'Til Health Do Us Part

'Til Health Do Us Part

One Woman's Extraordinary Story of Healing

Julie Rooney

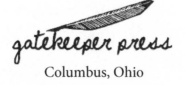

gatekeeper press

Columbus, Ohio

'Til Health Do Us Part

Copyright © 2018 by Julie Rooney

ISBN (hardcover): 9781642373721
ISBN (paperback): 9781642373738
eISBN: 9781642373745

Printed in the United States of America

To every woman who has lost hope and
is struggling to find it again,
I dedicate this book.

Contents

Every journey has a beginning. My journey to health began with illness, and you can't understand one without the other. So, I've made every effort to accurately recount my experiences based on my journals and medical records, along with my own admittedly hazy memories. I've also left out certain details, and have changed the names of my husband and our children, so that in telling my story I won't force them to tell theirs. Suffice it to say that we all struggled in our own ways, first with my getting sick and then with my getting well. And this story isn't about blame.

Prologue

THIS IS A story about healing. About *me* healing. And since my story is such a dramatic one, a lot of people have insisted on calling it a miracle. But it wasn't. At least not according to me, even though the changes in my outward appearance were so striking that people who got to know me when I was sick didn't recognize me after I'd healed. They'd literally walk right past me. Not that you could *see* what the matter was with me when I was sick. All you could see was what the medications had done to me.

And yet there was *something* miraculous about my journey from illness to health, at least to the extent that all change begins with some kind of prayer and seems to require some sort of divine energy. But whether or not my healing was miraculous, it certainly didn't occur overnight. I needed a year and a half to heal. And I had to do it on my own.

Well, not exactly on my own. I had a guide. But of course I couldn't just follow in his footsteps. That would have been too easy. Instead, I had to find my own path, like everyone else has to find theirs. I had to learn how to heal *myself*. Or better yet I had to learn how to *allow* myself to heal. And I couldn't do that until I was able to accept an almost unbearable truth.

That I too bore responsibility for what had happened to me.

Along the way I also had to change my thinking about the roots of disease, about the way I nourished myself and about the way toxic emotional environments can affect our health. Only then could I heal. And not just physically.

That said, I should warn you that my story's not a pretty one, and

1

the part I played in it wasn't always pretty. But it happened just the same.

I went through more than ten years of medical treatments, surgeries and procedures. Years that left me bloated, dazed and stripped of hope. To say nothing of the exhaustion that came from raising four kids while my husband traveled almost non-stop. And from the heartache that came from watching each one of my children land in trouble of one kind or another as my illnesses advanced. Even though I'd followed my doctors' orders and had gone along with every treatment my medical team proposed.

I have the medical correspondence to prove it.

And why wouldn't I have gone along with the treatment my doctors proposed? I was a registered nurse and my husband was a physician. A physician who worked for a major pharmaceutical company based in Silicon Valley, and one who'd earned a global reputation for his work in anti-viral therapies. A man who had saved many lives, and made a lot of money.

But this is *my* story, and I wrote it for two reasons.

First, because I needed to come to grips with what happened to me. And I figured the best way to do that was to write the story down. So I did, with the help of several writing workshops, two writers, an editor and many of my closest friends. The whole process, in fact, took a couple years longer than it did for me to heal.

Second, miracle or not, if reading this book convinces just one other woman out there that she can heal too, then all the trouble and the heartache and the hard work will have been worth it.

My story begins in the summer of 2010. At the time, as a side effect of the synthetic steroids I was taking, I weighed almost two hundred pounds. I was being treated for a laundry list of auto-immune diseases and was taking dozens of pills a day. And that's not counting injections and IVs.

My forty-ninth birthday was just a few months away, and no one was making any plans for my fiftieth.

Part I
Leaving

Chapter One

THE REALIZATION FINALLY comes to me on a quiet summer evening in northern California.

I can't do this anymore.

I'm sitting on a deck chair next to my husband, Rob. Our two youngest children, Cole and Catherine, are sitting to his right talking about who knows what. Cole is twenty, and Catherine's eighteen. Our oldest son, Liam, is twenty-six, and lives thousands of miles away in Hawaii. Nathan, our second born, is twenty-five. He's hanging out somewhere with his friends.

I think.

All of the chairs are drawn up around the fire pit but somehow I still feel like I'm on the outside. Rob has a glass of red wine cupped in one hand. The kids are holding glasses too, and it's a sure thing they're not filled with water. My eyes fall on Catherine, our youngest, whom we call Cat. Hard to believe how tall she is. How grown up and beautiful. Especially after the toll my last ten years took on all of us. Seems like she was a little girl just a few years ago, and yet she's starting college in the fall.

Well. I swore I'd get them all through high school. And now I have. Whether I'll see all of them graduate from college is another thing.

The warm summer air is thick with the scent of roses. Hundreds of them are in bloom on the hillside in front of us. Almost too beautiful to be real. Reds, whites, yellows, purples and pinks. Bold brushstrokes of color. I had them planted when we first moved in.

How many years is it now? Ten? Twelve?

Whatever.

Back then I still had the strength and the energy to manage a project like that. To supervise the gardeners as they buried irrigation lines in the hard earth. Dug holes for the bushes and spread mulch over the hill. The roses were for Rob. Because Rob loves roses and I love Rob and grand dramatic gestures are my thing.

Or *were* my thing.

Today I could care less.

"This ship has sunk," I say, more to myself than to anyone else.

Cat and Cole stop talking. They know what I mean. And so does Rob. He gives me the old you-know-how-the-steroids-affect-your-thinking look. If he didn't have a wine glass in his hand, he'd probably pat me on the arm.

How I hate that look. Like I can't be trusted anymore. Like I'm someone or some*thing* to be pitied. I look into his eyes and with a strength born of desperation, I hold his gaze. "I mean it. I can't do this anymore."

I try to control my voice because I want him to know that I'm serious. That I'm in my right mind. But my medications make it hard for me to talk sometimes, so all I can do is hope I'm not slurring my words.

Rob sighs. He's seen this show before. Me out on the ledge. But always looking back. Hoping he'll pull me away. And things will be all right again. Like they used to be.

My endocrinologist, who I'd seen earlier that week, doesn't share that hope. "You're between a rock and a hard place," she told me as gently as she could. "If the drugs don't kill you, your diseases will."

Not disease. Diseases.

Beginning in April of 2000 I'd been diagnosed with the first of three autoimmune diseases collectively known as Polyglandular Autoimmune Syndrome Type II—Addison's disease, Type I Diabetes and Hypothyroidism. On top of that, I had also been diagnosed with metastatic Crohn's, another autoimmune condition. And with the diseases came the drugs.

Prednisone, Dexamethasone, Cortef, Florinef and DHEA to manage the Addison's. Insulin for the diabetes. Enbrel, followed by Remicade, and then Humira for the Crohn's. Levoxyl for the hypothyroidism. And then there were the drugs I needed to offset the side effects of the primary medications. Lipitor for high cholesterol. Trilipix for high triglycerides. Forteo to help with the osteoporosis caused by the steroids used to treat the Addison's.

There was only one escape from the endless appointments and lab tests and let's-see-if-this-works cocktail of medications. Not to mention the crippling depressions, which at times made my physical complaints seem almost manageable.

With my endocrinologist's words still ringing in my ears I consoled myself with the thought that at least I don't have to go out and buy a gun. All I have to do is stop taking my medications and let my diseases finish me off. Or keep taking them and let the side effects do me in.

Rob and the kids have lost count of the number of times I've *nearly* died over the past ten years. So that afternoon, when I tell Cat and Cole and Rob that I've really had it, the words fall flat, exhausted from overuse. The kids glance at each other and then wait for a beat to see if I have anything else to say. I don't, and they go back to their conversation, keeping their voices low.

Which hurts, of course. Like it always does. But I can't really blame them. After ten years of sitting in the front row of my ongoing medical drama they're exhausted.

I shift my weight uncomfortably in the patio chair and wait for Rob to respond, hoping he'll tell me that everything's going to be all right. That we'll get through this like we've gotten through everything else. That he doesn't want me to give up because we still have a lot to live for.

He says nothing.

9

I reach for my cane and tap the top of the walking cast that envelops my right foot, trying to relieve an itch. It's the seventh cast I've had in fourteen months. This one's for a fractured 5th metatarsal. A few weeks ago I opened the car door and stepped out onto the driveway and the bone simply snapped. Just like that. Like a muffled gunshot. The time before that I was pushing my shopping cart down the aisle. The time before that I tripped over our dog's bed.

At forty-eight I have the bone density of an eighty-five-year-old woman.

"I think I'm going to fly over to Oahu with Cat," I say. "Maybe a change of scene will do me some good."

Rob clears his throat. "Just do whatever you need to do to get well."

The words sting as if he'd slapped me and I blink back tears. There *is* no prognosis for me getting well and he knows that. I shift my bulk in the chair. Try to find a position that's less uncomfortable and wonder just what it is I'm going to do if I can't do *this* anymore.

The kids chatter away. Rob sips his wine. To the west, the sinking sun leaves purple and blue bruises on the clouds.

Chapter Two

God I'm tired. Tired all the time now. Tired of telling everyone what I think they want to hear. Tired of telling my doctors and my husband that I'll do whatever they say. Tired of acting like something good is going to come of it. Tired of the grind mostly. I can't breathe here anymore. I need to get away. Need to clear my head. And flying to Oahu with our daughter to help get her set up at the beach house will have to do for now.

Cat is about to start her first year at Hawaii Pacific University. In Honolulu. She's going to live with Cole in one of the houses we own on Kaneohe Bay, about ten miles east of the city. The kids and I spent a lot of time there before I got sick. Rob would fly in to join us for a few days whenever he could. But that was before my illnesses made traveling so hard for me. And for everyone else too. But I've decided to go over with Cat anyway, and help her get settled for school. Maybe see Aliceanne and Francesca. Get some deep body massage or acupuncture. Stay a week or two.

While I pack a bag, Cat stretches out on the other side of the bed Rob and I share and starts flipping through a magazine. I glance at her, and for just a moment see the two-year-old girl who quit drinking milk from a bottle before her older brother Cole did. Just waved the bottle away one morning and reached for a cup. A little girl who was always in control. Or always trying to be.

"It's okay if you fly over with me," she says, "but I'm not gonna be able to take care of you once we get there. I'm gonna be *really* busy at school."

She's right about that. Especially because she's going to have to take a bus to get to her classes. On account of the DUI she picked up right after she turned eighteen.

"Don't worry, I can take care of myself," I say, pressing a neatly folded stack of clothes into my suitcase.

We're both saying the right things but I know she's worried about me interfering with her life. Not whether I'll be alive for Christmas. And I can't really blame her.

Tears well up in my eyes. "Just remember, sweetheart," I say, "No matter what happens, I'll always . . ."

". . . I *know*, Mom . . . you'll always be there for me."

"Well, it's true," I say, my voice cracking. "I will be. Even when . . ."

". . . *Mom*, I get it," she says, her eyes still on the magazine. "You must've told us a thousand times. But I still don't see why you're making *such* a big deal out of it now. Just keep taking your meds."

She sounds just like Rob. In fact, she sounds like all my doctors. Okay, maybe not *all* of them. Not my endocrinologist anyway. But the rest of them must have seen the writing on the wall too. They just won't read it out loud. Some sort of professional code of honor, I guess.

Never let them know there's no hope.

I shake a nightie out, and as I refold it to tuck it into my suitcase, I can't help thinking that two of me could have fit into it the day Rob and I were married. Then, still holding the flimsy thing in my hands, my thoughts drift to another item of intimate wear and another suitcase.

Rob's suitcase. From just a few weeks ago.

He had just gotten home but had to leave again the following morning. Which isn't unusual. These days he comes and goes so often he doesn't even unpack. Just unzips his suitcase and drapes it over the green chaise in our bedroom. Anyway, that afternoon, looking for laundry to fill out a load, I found an unfamiliar pair of black women's panties in his zippered suitcase pocket.

12

"They must be Cat's," he said when I confronted him, dangling the underwear from one of my fingers. "Ada probably got them mixed up in the laundry."

When I didn't respond Rob gave me the old look. The look he always gave me if I raised the issue of infidelity. "Sweetheart, you know the steroids make you paranoid."

As a nurse I knew he was right. Psychosis is one of the side effects of regular corticosteroid use. And yet as I stood there with that strange woman's panties swinging from my finger, I didn't feel the least bit psychotic. I felt wounded. Cheated on. Lied to.

I may be sick, but I'm a woman who knows her family's underwear.

Part II
Waiting

Chapter Three

THE LAST DAYS of the summer of 2010 slip away like sand through my fingers. Not that anything actually changes here on Oahu. September is just as beautiful as August, when Cat and I flew in. October will be just as beautiful as September. I feel like I'm between seasons myself. Not living, not dying. Stuck between the rock of my illnesses and the hard place of my medications.

Cat has settled into the rental house with Cole. He's studying at Hawaii Pacific too. So our two youngest are only a few minutes away. Liam and his girlfriend Allison live in the yellow house, right across the driveway. I live in the white house.

By myself.

I hate to be alone, and for some reason I think back to how Liam hated to be alone too. Had terrible separation anxiety as a child. In fact it got so bad that when I started dropping him off at preschool I had to use tricks to calm him down.

"Listen, sweetie," I'd whisper, pressing an old car key into his tiny hand. "You hold on to this key and then I'll *have* to come back here to get you. You know, 'cause the car can't start if I don't have a key."

"Okay, mommy," he'd respond, wide-eyed, looking up at me like what I'd just told him was the most important thing in the whole world. "I'm puttin' this key in my pocket right now."

As silly as it sounds, it worked. In fact, it worked so well that there are days I find myself wishing somebody would give *me* a car key.

I'm just not used to being by myself. Not after twenty-seven years of marriage and four kids. And I have *way* too much time to think about it. It doesn't help that each day is exactly the same. That each day passes with the same mind-numbing regularity. Like a pendulum swinging back and forth, and back and forth, underneath a broken clock.

Wake up, test my blood sugar, fill my insulin pump, attach my insulin pump, and check my blood pressure. Swallow a handful of pills, adjust my steroids, worry that the Crohn's is inhibiting the absorption of the steroids and wonder if I will descend into diabetic shock. Adjust my insulin pump, wondering all the while, will today be the day my blood sugar spikes and I collapse? The day my blood pressure drops so low that I just keel over?

I've been thinking about flying back to California now that Cat's started school. But what's the point? Liam, Cole and Cat are here on the island. Nathan's at school in Colorado. And Rob's in Europe. I think. Or maybe it's South Africa. I can't remember, but it doesn't really matter. If I can't reach him, my doctors are just a phone call away. In the meantime, my diseases and the drugs can fight it out to see who gets me first.

I decide to call my son. "Hi Nathan, it's Mom. Just callin' to see how you're doin'." I pause, not wanting to leave such a short message, I guess because I want to give him a chance to pick up. And besides, just like always, I don't have *any* idea what I'm going to say to his answering machine, even though I know I'm probably going to be talking to *it*, not Nathan.

"It's a . . . beautiful day here on the island . . . hope it's not too cold in Colorado. Which reminds me, your dad and I were kind of hoping you're *not* gonna fall into another frozen pond this year. Just stay inside when you're drinking, okay? You know, when it's cold out."

I imagined he was probably snoring away in the middle of the day. Sleeping one off. Or just lying there listening to me, with no intention whatsoever of picking up the phone. I wait a moment. "Well, okay. Hope *you're* okay, and, you know, you're getting to all your classes."

Fat chance of that.

"And don't worry about me, I'm doin' fine. Just have to keep an eye on my blood sugar . . . you know, and the dexamethasone . . . but you don't need to hear about all of that."

I'm sure if you asked him he'd say he never really *needed* to hear about any of my medications again. "Okay, Nathan. Talk to you later. Love you."

I sit next to the phone for another minute or so, but Nathan calling me back was about as likely as Publisher's Clearinghouse calling to say I'd won the big prize.

Yeah, I'm whining again, I know. But by now it's as fixed a part of my routine as checking my blood sugar. In fact I'm beginning to wonder if whining isn't an underreported side effect of synthetic steroids.

The only time I do anything different is when my bloodwork changes. Most of the time I just sit out on the lanai, looking across Kaneohe Bay and sipping my tea. Thinking back over all the decisions I've made, good and bad, and all the people who've been in my life. I know. It's probably a waste of time. But looking back is so much easier than looking ahead. And in this state of limbo the past seems closer somehow. As if I can turn and see it sitting there right next to me.

When I was a little girl we always ate dinner as a family. Even if my dad had gone into town and come back late, we always sat down to eat together. My mom gave each of us something to do while she got dinner ready. Somebody had to set the table. Somebody else had to shuck the corn. The dogs had to be fed. Glasses of milk had to be poured. And everything had to be done by the time my dad got home or we were in big trouble.

I can still see the five of us gathered around the dinner table. Our hands are folded in front of us. My head is bowed and my eyes are closed. My legs swing slightly in the space beneath my chair. Metronomes out of sync. I am five years old.

It's my turn to say grace, but I can't remember the first words.

God is. No. That's not it.

At first my father is impatient, but as the seconds tick past, anger rises off him like heat from an oven. Everyone else feels it too, but they just sit there while I squeeze my eyes tighter and tighter and try to get the words out. My heart flutters in my chest like a hummingbird in a cage.

Thank you for the. No that's not right.

My mother clears her throat and my sister Beth draws in a deep breath. My father seems to grow larger, until his head and shoulders throw a shadow over our small kitchen table. Tears burn in the corners of my eyes. Everyone's dinner is getting cold and it's my fault.

The legs of my dad's chair scrape back against the floor and a calloused hand grabs me by the back of my neck. My mother, sister and brother don't take their eyes off their plates.

Run.

I pull away and bolt toward the stairs, but my father is too fast. His hand shoots out again and grabs hold of me. Behind me, I hear his belt buckle clink, and then I hear the whisper of leather as he pulls his belt through the loops of his khaki pants.

Chapter Four

IT SEEMS LIKE I'm never really hungry anymore. Not since I got to Oahu anyway. I eat just to keep my insulin levels stable. Take steroids when my blood pressure drops. Wrap my cast in a plastic bag with a blue plastic ring to keep the water out when I shower. Change my insulin pump and pray for courage.

Or for an infection they can't treat.

Whining. I know.

Every four or five days I call my endocrinologist just to let her know I'm still alive. Wait a minute or two for her secretary to put me through while twirling the telephone cord around one finger. "Good morning, Julie. How're you feeling?"

"Pretty good, I guess."

"How's your blood sugar?"

"It's a little low."

"Okay. Sounds like we should take another look at your dexamethasone dosage. Are you still in Hawaii?"

"Yeah, I'm still here."

"Well, let me know when you're going to be back in California, and if you have to see anyone in the meantime, have them send the blood work to us."

"Okay. Thanks again for everything."

"You're welcome, Julie. Just wish I could do more for you."

But she can't. In fact none of them can. So, most of the time I just sit on the lanai and look out over the water. Or go back inside to watch HGTV. When it's dark, I crawl into bed and curl up in the fetal position and wait for sleep. But sleep doesn't come. Just memories.

Of the small farm in Maryland, where I grew up. My father worked and my mother took care of the house and the kids. She put meals on the table too and somehow found time to help Dad with the chickens and the garden and the bookkeeping.

In the summer my little brother David and I collected green Coke bottles from the side of the road and traded them at the little local store for penny candy. We brought in as many bottles as we could carry and left the store with Mary Janes, Squirrel Nut Zippers, Sweet Tarts and Root Beer Barrels stuffed into our pockets. Pushing through the old screen door, we ran past the old men who sat on the covered porch telling stories and laughing at things we didn't understand.

Every fall we had to go back to school, but nobody acted like it really mattered. It was just what kids had to do. Listen to the teacher and do your homework. But even the kids who graduated from high school ended up back on the farm. Unless they were lucky and found a job in Ocean City.

My dad's father, my grandfather, was born in Hungary. My grandma told me once the only thing he ever really wanted to do his whole life was get to America. And once he got here, she said, all he wanted to do was sit around and drink beer. Pabst Blue Ribbon. My father was different. He earned his plumber's license and his electrician's license and he finally got his general contractor's license too.

"And they don't give those out to just anybody," he'd tell us at the dinner table.

Chapter Five

ROB AND I try to talk every day. Or at least I try to talk to him every day. But he's pretty busy. Hard to get a hold of, especially from the middle of the Pacific ocean. Always in a meeting or at a conference or on his way to a business dinner. And not only in a different time zone but sometimes half a day away. So when I worry that it's Monday and he hasn't called, it turns out that it's already Tuesday wherever he is.

So I sit near the phone a lot. Waiting for him to return my calls. But just like a watched pot never boils, a watched phone never rings.

And when he finally does call he never has time to talk. "Hi, honey. Everything all right?"

"Yeah, yeah, everything's good," I say, my mind still half asleep after sitting there watching the phone for hours. "Where are you?"

"Jules, come on. I told you I was in Hong Kong."

"Oh yeah, now I remember."

"Kids all right?"

"The kids? Yeah, I guess so. I don't really see that much of . . ."

". . . no, of course you don't. They're in school, where they should be."

"Yeah, guess you're right," I reply, desperately trying to remember why I wanted to talk to him. "Look, do you have any idea when . . ."

"...Julie, I'm late for breakfast, so I've gotta run. Give me a call tomorrow if you have a chance."

If I have a chance. What does he think I'm doing here?

More memories crowd back into the present. Like the day I found out that my older sister Beth wasn't my dad's real daughter. The truth was in an old letter in the bottom of a drawer in my Mom's desk. I can't remember what I was looking for, but I don't think I moved for a long time after I read it. Like my world was a shoebox, and we were all toys inside it. And somebody had just turned it upside down and started shaking it.

The thing was I couldn't ask anybody about it, because if they'd kept it a secret all those years they certainly wouldn't tell me now. But over the years I put the pieces together. My mother had married Beth's dad when she was fifteen. Two years later Beth was born, but the marriage didn't work out. I think there was something wrong with him. Anyway, after my father and mother got married he adopted Beth. And he didn't just give her a new last name, he changed her first name too. She used to be called Yvonne.

So my parents lied to me and David all those years. Or at the very least, they didn't tell us the truth. We thought things were one way when they were really another.

Beth was six years older than I was. My dad used the belt on her all the time. And my mother told her over and over again that if a girl wasn't careful she could get into trouble. I didn't know what kind of trouble my mom was talking about, although I was pretty sure it wasn't the sort of trouble a little girl could get into. But Beth didn't listen. She kept doing whatever she wanted to do, like staying out late, and she never backed down. Not even after my dad knocked her out of her chair and fractured one of her vertebrae.

Sometimes I felt so sorry for her I'd sneak her tea and toast after she'd been grounded and sent to her room. Not that she'd ever thank me. In fact once, in a fit of spite, she took the plate and the cup from me and then told me I was adopted. "Dad's best friend, Richie, is your real father," she said.

I was only ten, but I knew it wasn't true. She was just blaming me for the way my dad treated her. Which meant I still had to take care of her. Because that's just the way it was. You had to earn love in our family. You had to do what your dad and mom told you to do. You had to think about everybody else first. Not yourself.

Chapter Six

I F TIME IS all life gives us, then I'm rich. Because I have all the time in the world. But I don't have a thing to do with it. Or more accurately, I can't *do* anything with it, because I can barely hobble from one end of the house to the other. So I sit around and think about what might have been.

After a decade of chronic illnesses, that's what I do. Worry that I won't live. Worry that I will. Not sure which frightens me more.

Rob has flown over a couple of times. His visits never last more than a few days. We go shopping at Costco. Sit on the lanai in the afternoon and stare at the bay. Neither of us knows what to say. We sleep in the same bed but we don't make love.

We don't talk about how Rob can't stand to touch me anymore.

And yet there is some small part of me that still hopes things will change. That thinks spending a little time apart will end up bringing us together again. But it's not working out that way. Instead, I just get that sinking feeling in the pit of my stomach. One I know far too well.

The next day Rob flies off again and that afternoon I get into another argument with my neighbor. He owns the house next door, which has been turned into three or four apartments, and he's always complaining about something. "Your son *never* cleans up after his dog, and there are flies everywhere," he complains to me.

27

He's right. All the properties along the bay kind of blend into one as they hit the beach, and Liam's dog Buddha does his business whenever he feels the urge, no matter whose house he's in front of.

"Well," I say, trying to buy time, "I'll tell him again. As soon as I see him."

"As soon as you see him? He lives right next to you. And while you're at it would you tell him to turn the garage light out at night, too? It shines right into my bedroom."

"I'll let him know."

"And would it kill him to mow your lawns more than once a month? You guys are driving down property values around here."

"You know I'd do it myself if I could . . ."

". . . but you can't, which is why *he* should be doing it."

This goes on for a while longer. The garbage cans are always overflowing. Loud music late at night. Beer cans everywhere. Cars parked on the front lawn. Can't really argue with him. The description is so accurate you could find the place without a street number.

I first began to develop gastrointestinal problems in high school. While other girls filled out, I lost weight. Got kidney stones. Not that anyone else seemed to notice what was going on. Instead, by the time I was sixteen, boys and men were staring at me openly as I went by. The boys flirted and the men asked me out on dates. My parents saw what was going on. After all, they'd just been through it with Beth. So, they didn't say no, they just encouraged me to entertain "older" boys. Of course, that would be older boys from the "right" families. By the time I turned seventeen, I'd spent more than one weekend away with a boy masquerading as a man, compromising myself to please him. But I was really doing it to please my parents, who wanted me to find someone to take me off their hands. Just like Beth had. But I still enjoyed the attention and the pleasure of being with a man.

"What we tried with your sister didn't work," my father told me. "So you do what you want, just as long as you don't ruin my good name."

What I wanted? The thought hadn't entered my mind for years.

Everything I did, and everything I'd ever done, seemed to be a transaction of some kind or another. Just another entry in the family ledger, hopefully on the plus side. Something to balance the violence. The craziness. My father sitting on the back stairs, his head in his hands, threatening suicide. Or my mother holding a pewter bowl high in the air as he sat at the kitchen table, telling him she'd hit him over the head with it if he didn't stop.

In the spring of '79, the year I graduated from high school, I was going out with a boy named Danny. Lean, good-looking, and with a full head of curly hair, he wasn't exactly from one of the "right" families. But he was a year older than I was, and he owned his own tow truck. And that summer he was starting to make some real money. At least for a nineteen-year-old. And since I'd told myself I was in love with him, I went along for the ride. But we both knew that when the summer was over, so were we.

I had to do something with my life. I'd never been much of a student, so teaching was out. And I couldn't type, so secretarial work wasn't in my future either. That left nursing. So following in my sister's footsteps, I made plans to enroll in a two-year nursing program that fall.

Chapter Seven

THE HOURS CRAWL by like bugs making the long trek across the lanai. I'm not used to the slow pace. Or at least I didn't used to be.

When I graduated from nursing school, at nineteen, I went right to work as a trauma nurse. Didn't even think of it as work. I liked moving quickly to keep a patient alive. Applying tourniquets. Charging the defibrillators.

Now I spend my time crocheting blankets for my grown children. Just to have something to do. To keep me in the now. But it doesn't work. You can't crochet illness away. So I let my mind wander. Anything to keep my mind off the present.

When I first laid eyes on Rob, in the summer of 1980, I'd never have guessed that he'd be the man I'd spend the next thirty-four years of my life with. I was filling in for one of the nurses at a walk-in clinic on the Ocean City boardwalk and he just happened to be covering for one of the doctors.

He was wearing a clean dress shirt and dress pants beneath his white lab coat, but because of the heat, I guess, was wearing sandals instead of dress shoes. He had deep blue eyes and thick dark hair that ran back across his head in waves. And even though his mustache seemed designed to hide a baby face, it was easy to see that he was older than me. But then again, every doctor was.

When he asked me what I was doing later I told him I was already going out with someone. "I don't care," he said.

He smiled easily, I had to give him that. And he had a self-confidence about him. Or maybe he was just stubborn. No matter how hard I tried, I couldn't put him off. He just followed me around all night but in a casual, self-assured sort of way. And rare for a physician, when he asked me a question it almost seemed as if he listened to my answer.

A few days later he got his hands on the schedule and started showing up whenever I was working. After successfully prying my number out of me, he even called my house and introduced himself to my mother. "I'm still going out with Danny," I said when she told me he had called.

"But Rob's a doctor," said Mom.

She was right. He was a doctor. And he was tall and good looking too. To say nothing of being well-educated and cultured. Like no one I'd ever known. And he talked to me about things no one else ever had. Had a wild side too. He liked to stay up all night, drink good wine, and jump into the hot tub naked. His friends from medical school did too. The whole bunch of them partied every night, did drugs, and peeled out of their clothes as soon as they got to the beach.

Which made me a little uncomfortable. I was used to drinking Miller ponies and taking an occasional drag on a joint. Used to riding around in pickup trucks or GTOs and making love in the middle of cornfields. And they were all much older than I was. But their wildness was infectious, and so, that August, I probably slept on the sand more often than I slept in a bed. And lying there on the beach at night, staring up into the stars and listening to the waves crash against the shore, I couldn't help thinking about Beth. Who got a beating whenever she didn't come home at night.

"Just don't ruin my good name," was all my father had said.

By the middle of the summer Danny and the tow truck were history, and Rob was the future.

Chapter Eight

OUR FAMILY PHOTO albums are all back in California. But sitting here in Kaneohe Bay with so much time on my hands I often feel like I've got one of them open in my lap. Like I'm leafing through the images in my mind.

There I am when I was still young, healthy and beautiful.

Rob and I when we still had a chance.

The kids when they were bright-eyed and happy.

Every time I go inside, I stop in front of the hall mirror. Hoping to see me as I was. But that me is never there. And I hardly recognize the old, overweight, defeated woman looking out at me. So I go back outside. Settle into my chair and wait.

And wait.

Some days running out of cigarettes is the only thing that gets me out of the house. The supermarket's not far, just right up the road, but it's a bit of a production to get out of the house and into the car when you're in a walking cast. Which I am most of the time.

"All this stuff yours?" says the checkout guy, glancing at the woman in line behind me.

"Yeah, sorry," I say, reaching for one of those little black bars that lets them know whose stuff is whose.

The guy drags two loaves of white bread, a squeeze bottle of mustard, two pounds of smoked turkey, a couple of six-packs of diet soda and two packages of dessert cakes across the scanner, which beeps every time it reads one of the items.

"Let me have a couple packs of Winstons, too," I say as the conveyor belt stops and he reaches for the heavy black bar back behind my stuff.

"Hard pack or soft?"

"Soft, please."

When I'm not crocheting blankets or crying in front of the HGTV or tending to my endless medical needs, I go outside and sneak a cigarette. Chain-drink Diet Cokes and watch the rain descend over the mountains. I know I'm not supposed to be smoking. Or drinking so much caffeine either. But it's not like quitting is going to make a difference this late in the game. Which makes me think back to some of the more difficult patients I had when I started out as a nurse. When I couldn't understand why everyone didn't just follow the doctors' orders.

Who did they think they were?

Rob grew up in Massachusetts. Just outside of Boston. But after his father was transferred to Maryland, he stayed behind and moved in with his elderly Aunt Florence. His parents didn't want to interrupt his education at the prestigious prep school he was attending.

The family's decision paid off big time. In 1970, he was accepted into Harvard. Four years later he started medical school. When I met him in 1980, he had just finished his residency and was studying for his boards in internal medicine and infectious diseases. And finishing up a research project he'd started in medical school. He had plans to travel to Pakistan at the end of the summer. Something to do with gathering field data for his project.

So he took off for the other side of the world and I went back to college to finish my associate degree in nursing. Got postcards from him every now and then. Flowers, too. Big gaudy bouquets of carnations, I guess because they were the cheapest. The smell always made me think of funerals, but of course I never told Rob that.

34

Back on the lanai, I light up a cigarette and look out over the bay. Take in the way the glittering turquoise shallows give way to the deeper blue farther offshore. Squint at the dark green cliffs of the Ko'olau range rising in the distance. Towering over the tranquil water.

Not really a mountain range at all. Just what's left of the crater formed by some ancient volcano. Which is all my present really is. The remnants of my past.

By the end of my last year in nursing school, walking into a hospital lobby had begun to feel like coming home. This was the place I'd been trained to live and work in for the rest of my life. The world of Western medicine. Of light green linoleum floors and beige walls. Of doctors in white lab coats, stethoscopes dangling from their necks, and clipboards in hand, striding through the halls like demigods. Hard-to-understand announcements coming from ceiling speakers. Muted-colored curtains hung from noisy curtain rods that separated the two beds in each room. The smell of cleanliness. Of chemical sterility. Occasionally overridden by the flowers in the patients' rooms.

By the time Rob got back from Pakistan, I'd already graduated. I had a job at the local hospital and had rented a small apartment.

And then one night he just showed up at my door.

Chapter Nine

WHEN DEPRESSION FOGS me in, I stump my way back into the house, open the refrigerator and make sure that the insulin I hid behind the baking soda is still there. Way more than enough to *accidentally* administer a fatal overdose. If it comes to that. Death by miscalculation of insulin. Happens all the time to diabetics. No one would be the wiser.

But who am I kidding? I can't bear the thought of one of my children showing up at the house and finding my lifeless body on the couch. Especially if they knew I'd died by my own hand. Couldn't hang that on them too.

Cole calls to tell me he's not going to make it for lunch. Like I don't know that, since I've already called him six or seven times, and it's after 2:30 now.

"I'm not feeling so good, Mom." I'm about to tell him I'm not feeling so good either, but decide against it. Even though I'm the one who's sick, not him. And I'm not the one drinking so much that I'm flunking out of school again, either. I'd go over there if it weren't for my walking cast. I would. At least that way his dog Maya would get fed.

In 1981, I began to show early signs of arthritis. At first the doctors thought it was carpal tunnel, but when they opened my right wrist

37

up surgically, they found an arthritic nodule. The rheumatologist I consulted a few months later told me she couldn't be sure, but she thought the arthritis was an early manifestation of some sort of autoimmune disease. If I wanted children, the pregnancies might be difficult.

Rob and I weren't engaged at the time. We weren't even living together. But he knew how important having children was to me. In fact, I'd talked about it on our first date in Ocean City.

"So, what do you want to do with your life?" he'd asked me, just to start a conversation, I think. After considering my answer for a few seconds I decided I'd just tell him the truth.

"I want to get married and have five boys."

He spit his drink out and choked.

So he knew. Right from the beginning. And he knew why too.

I wanted a chance to break the cycle. To raise my family differently. Without the craziness and the violence and all the other stuff I'd never be able to forget. And since the doctor said I was on borrowed time where having kids was concerned, there was no time to waste.

The morning after I saw the rheumatologist, Rob kissed me, told me to have a good day, and left for work. When he got home that night he said he had an announcement to make. "We're getting married."

Chapter Ten

Rob continues to fly in and out of Hawaii. Sometimes he comes from the East, sometimes from the West. The children keep their distance, angry that I seem to have given up.

"Do you think that people can have sex just for fun?" he asks me, out of the blue. I haven't thought about having fun for years. Or sex. All I think about is staying alive.

The next day he's gone again.

Or was it two days?

My medications make me lose track of the days. The years begin to swim together too, and sometimes I can't even remember when Rob and I first met. Or when we were married. The meds have taken those memories.

I call Cat.

"Mom, I can't talk now. If I miss the bus, I'm gonna be late for work."

I'll give her credit for that. She's the only one of our kids who works. At Pinky's, this pupu bar and grill just outside the Marine base. And she has to take the bus to get there.

"Okay, honey, I'll call back later."

"How about tomorrow, mom? My classes don't start until late. Maybe you could even give me a ride."

In the spring of 1983, after we announced our engagement, Rob and his mother and I went out to look for an engagement ring. She insisted that I pick out something fancy. I chose a small, antique rose-cut diamond ring instead. By then it was too late in the year to book any of the best wedding spots. So, we decided we'd just get married as soon as we could, wherever we could.

We invited over two hundred guests, from over twenty states and six different countries. I didn't know most of them, but Rob had made a lot of friends and worked with a lot of people over the course of his education. The guests filled two hotels. The ceremony was held in a Catholic Church at the southern tip of a barrier island, not ten miles away from the farm on which I'd been raised. There was no Mass, just an eighteen-minute traditional ceremony. Before it began, when the whole wedding party was just outside the church waiting to go in, Rob leaned down and whispered in my ear. "Don't forget, Julie, I'm Catholic, and Catholics don't believe in divorce."

Chapter Eleven

A s the days on Oahu go by, I think more and more about dying. At least I'd be at peace.

And to be honest, death *is* starting to look better and better. Not only because my body is failing, and bound to get worse. But also because living means I'll have to exist with the massive train wreck my life has become. I'll have to own up to the fact that my family has fallen apart. That my children are out of control. That my husband has been unfaithful. And that none of them have any respect for me.

Which isn't surprising, since I don't even respect myself anymore.

Continuing to live would also mean facing up to the fact that I've failed at the only thing I ever really wanted to do. That is, to give my kids a better childhood than the one I had. A childhood free of fear. And lies. And of having to *earn* love, which is the same thing as being told you don't *deserve* it.

Out on the lanai again, I hear raucous laughter from across the driveway. Sounds like Liam has some friends over, and they're laughing at Bud. That's Liam's African gray parrot. Who's named for Liam's favorite beer. Or a bud of marijuana. The story changes all the time.

Bud doesn't like me. Whenever I'm there he drops to the floor, sneaks up behind me and pecks my toes. Takes the nail polish right off. And I think some of Liam's friends have been training him to say "fatso" whenever I come in the room. Bud says "pretty boy" too, but what he's famous for is imitating the sound of bong water gurgling as someone takes a hit. And then coughing. It really is pretty funny, and the local student newspaper even ended up featuring Bud in an article. With a complete description of the bong gurgling, of course, followed by the obligatory cough.

Talk about your higher education.

Once Rob and I were married we quickly established a mating season. I'd always get pregnant in the late spring or early summer, which meant that each of our four children was born in the six-week period from the middle of February to the end of March.

The first to arrive was Liam, who was born eleven months after our honeymoon in Europe. The rest of them were Deep Creek Lake babies. That's the lake in western Maryland where we vacationed every spring. Nathan was the first to be conceived there and was born eleven months after Liam. He was born in February, and of course, he would have been the exception to the birth window if he hadn't been two months premature. I gained very little weight while I carried him, and lost too much weight after he was born.

My doctors said stress was to blame.

42

Chapter Twelve

THE SLOW DAYS of Hawaiian paradise go on and on. And isn't this what heaven's supposed to be like? Or is it hell? Where nothing out of the ordinary happens. I don't feel better. I don't get worse. Rob doesn't call. The kids don't call either, or come over. And when he does, or they do, I bitch and complain. I can't stop myself.

I am at a complete loss. I don't know what to do. I don't know what's going to happen.

So I do what anyone in my situation would do.

I call my psychic.

Aliceanne doesn't answer either. Wonder if there's something wrong with my phone. Like it only accepts incoming calls. That would explain a lot.

I make myself a cup of tea, go outside again and stare out across the bay. The drugs are playing with my mind again, and for a moment I can't remember when Aliceanne Parker and I first met. I'm pretty sure it was on a visit to the island a couple years back. In 2008. But I can't be certain. All I know is that Liam and Allison were going to Hawaii Pacific at the time and that Aliceanne was scheduled to speak to one of Allison's classes about the interpretation of dreams.

"Do you want to listen in?" Allison asked me. "My professor says Aliceanne's a psychic too."

I'm almost always on time. In fact I pride myself on it. But of course that day I was late, and so I ended up missing most of Aliceanne's presentation. But I got a good look at her before the class came to an end. Pretty. Thin. Neither tall nor short. Penetrating eyes. Easy smile. Silver hair cut short, standing straight up on her head. Gave her an elfish look. Hard to tell how old she was since she radiated so much energy.

We spoke for a few minutes after class and exchanged numbers. It wasn't as if I needed to explain anything to her. In 2008, I was at my worst. One look told you all you needed to know about my physical condition. Before Aliceanne left the classroom, she gave me a big hug and told me to call her. We could set up a reading.

By 1985, the stress my doctors blamed for my troubled pregnancies was still building, and a lot of it had to do with money. Rob had gone to work for the National Institutes of Health, and while the job was prestigious, it didn't pay very well. And we'd just bought our first house, all twelve hundred square feet of it, just outside Washington, D.C. With two adults and two children to feed and clothe, to say nothing of a mortgage payment and Rob's school loans to pay off, we often turned to our credit cards to make ends meet.

Or as Rob used to say, we lived off love.

He was already working one overnight a week in the emergency room to bring in more money, but we still came up short month after month. So, we finally decided to open a walk-in clinic of our own. It was no small undertaking, even after Rob got two other doctors involved. A building had to be leased, and used medical equipment and office furniture had to be bought at auction. Permits had to be applied for. We had to hire a business manager, a receptionist, a full-time nurse, someone to handle billing and a lab and X-ray tech. Our share of the startup costs came to seventeen thousand dollars. It might as well have been seventeen million. Rob asked his parents for a loan, and I asked mine, but they couldn't help. And who could blame them? In 1985 seventeen thousand dollars was a lot of money. So Rob went to the one financial institution that never turned him down.

The bank of Aunt Margo.

His aunt loaned us $30,000, and Rob and I began working twelve-hour shifts every Saturday and Sunday at our newly opened walk-in clinic. And while Rob's parents hadn't been able to loan us the money we needed to open the clinic, they were willing to watch the kids for us. If they hadn't been able to look after Liam and Nathan on the weekends, we'd never have been able to pull it off. My mother helped out too, but since she and my dad were now almost three hours away, we had to meet halfway, at a Denny's just across Chesapeake Bay.

During the week, when we were all together at home, things were a little less frantic. But there were still four of us packed into a small, three-bedroom house, and one of the bedrooms wasn't much bigger than a closet. And there was only one bathroom. On the second floor. And Nathan had one eye that required extra medical attention.

Work and the boys weren't the only reasons I kept finding myself in exam rooms. I just couldn't gain any weight. I'd weighed a hundred pounds when Rob and I were married, and I still weighed a hundred pounds after Nathan was born. My doctors suspected an eating disorder and sent me to Washington Hospital Center for evaluation. Part of that evaluation included a psych workup. In the end, I was pronounced borderline anorexic. Actually, what they said was that some people eat when they're under stress, and other people don't eat when they're under stress. In other words, none of them knew what was going on.

The truth was, I just never really felt well again after our first two children were born. But what young mother does? Still, with the two of us working in the clinic every weekend, we managed to pay the loan back. With interest, as Aunt Margo would tell anyone in the family who'd listen.

Chapter Thirteen

I KEEP CALLING ALICEANNE, but she doesn't answer. So I have long phone calls with friends on the mainland. The kids stop by every once in a while. I have occasional, brief conversations with the people who work in the pharmacy or at the supermarket. And with Rob, whenever he flies across the Pacific and stops for the night.

Finally, Aliceanne picks up.

Once we've talked about my situation for a while, Aliceanne pauses, then speaks to me in her rich, full-throated voice. "Your life has always been about love. Maybe now's a good time to use that love to heal yourself."

She's not talking about adding more meds.

When the kids tell Rob that I've been speaking to Aliceanne again, he calls to tell me how gullible I am. I prefer to think of myself as open to new ideas. And I don't care what anyone says. Science and religion can't possibly hold *all* the answers.

Thirty-six hours after Nathan was born we opened a second clinic. Again, without Rob's parents and my parents, we could never have pulled it off. And after our second child was born it seemed like every moment of every day was spoken for. So when my obstetrician said that I probably wasn't going to be able to get pregnant again it didn't seem like such a terrible thing. Besides, no one was surprised. After all, the rheumatologist from Johns Hopkins had warned me back in '82 that the older I got, the more trouble I'd have getting pregnant.

We were too busy to give it much thought. Rob drove off to his office in D.C. every weekday morning. I stayed home and took care of the kids. Then on the weekends I dropped Liam and Nathan off with Rob's parents so we could both pull twelve-hour shifts at our clinics.

We told ourselves it wouldn't be like this forever. Eventually we'd open a private practice together and raise our kids and be there for his parents and my parents too. And despite both of us being so stressed out, our life was turning out more or less the way we'd imagined it.

With one or two small exceptions.

Like Rob telling me about a nurse in the ER who tried to kiss him when they all went out for a drink after work and telling him how she wanted to party with him. Of course when I brought it up again the following morning after he sobered up, he denied saying it.

Or the time I had a panic attack during a party we threw for his friends at work. It got so bad that I hid in the backyard and then made things even worse by watching the other doctors and their elegant wives laugh and touch each other. It was like they were playing. Like it meant nothing to them. I felt completely out of my element, intellectually and culturally. They were all so well-educated, beautiful and wealthy. I obviously didn't belong.

Still, standing there behind those bushes, I was somehow able to remind myself that Rob had chosen me. Had pursued me. Had married me. Had fathered children with me. But as I repeated that litany, a woman came into view and started flirting with him. Running polished nails down the front of his shirt. Kissing him lightly on the cheek. And from where I stood it seemed as if he was enjoying the attention.

Much later, after everyone had left, I listened silently as Rob yelled at me for embarrassing him by running off and hiding like that. And then told me I was crazy for believing there was something going on between him and that woman.

Crazy.

Chapter Fourteen

I SPEND A LOT of time on the lanai thinking about my marriage.

Okay. Rob and I have had a little trouble. In fact, we've had a lot of trouble, and for a long time, and a lot of that trouble came along as my health worsened, and my focus turned inward. But I still love him. Still want to slip into bed alongside him. Press my back against his belly and pull his arms around me until it feels as if the two of us are one. Despite my illnesses. Despite his continual absences. Despite having been left alone to raise four children. Despite my certainty that he's been unfaithful.

And so it rankles when he flies in and talks so casually about how sex and commitment aren't the same things. That sometimes sex can just be for fun. Almost recreational. Like a workout at the gym. And it makes sense, doesn't it, he asks me, given the shape my body is in? I get up on one elbow and stare at him, searching his eyes. See that he's serious. And realize that some small part of me even understands his logic. Which *really* hurts.

"You need to be more understanding," he said. "Not put so many conditions on love."

When I don't respond he leans in and kisses me gently on the forehead.

"I wasn't trying to upset you," he whispers. "You know you're the love of my life."

And then he gets up and goes to the bathroom. Leaving me in bed by myself.

The first four or five years of our marriage we never *talked* in bed. Except when one of us needed a breather. Or I was pregnant and near my due date.

Our third son, Cole, was born in February of 1990. If he had waited one more day he would have been born on his brother Nathan's fifth birthday. But our family still wasn't complete. At least not the way Rob saw it. He wanted a girl. And as if he had placed an order, our daughter Catherine was born in February of 1992.

Rob and I never had a budget. When we needed more money, we just worked harder. Still, by the time Cat was born it was obvious to both of us that Rob's salary at the National Institutes of Health was never going to cover our bills, clinics or no clinics. And having had four kids over a span of seven years, I was no longer able to help out financially. It would have cost as much to pay the babysitters as I could have made as a nurse. And besides I didn't bring children into the world to watch someone else raise them. Not even their grandparents. Our two oldest boys were in elementary school by then and there was just too much to do what with the two little ones at home. Too much laundry to do. Too many breakfasts and lunches to make. Too many dinners to cook and baths to run.

We'd been married nine years by then and I had just what I'd asked for. Okay, I was on my own with the kids all day and never really seemed to be able to catch my breath but what mother does? At least I had a partner who came home at night. Not a husband who lived on the road. A man who was part of the family. Not just a provider and an enforcer like my father was. Someone who only came home to be fed and to wash and to sleep and to have his clothes washed. Or to hit his children if they misbehaved.

All I wanted was a family and a husband who came home at night.

But who was I fooling? We both knew things had to change. Four young children in a tiny house with one bathroom? How was that going to work? And as long as Rob continued to work at the NIH, even with the extra income from the clinics, we'd never be able to afford a place big enough for all of us.

So, six months after Cat was born Rob took a job with a private biomedical research foundation in North Carolina. "You won't need to work," he told me. "I'll be making more in a day than you could make in a week."

And just like that my nursing career was over, even though I insisted on keeping my license current. Rob didn't fight me. Said it was a good idea. You could never tell.

Chapter Fifteen

"ROB AND YOUR children aren't doing anything wrong, darling," Aliceanne tells me when we speak again. "They're just living the lives they want to live, so don't waste your time blaming them. You need to look at yourself. Take responsibility for your own life."

The tears come on so fast I can't stop them.

"Don't you think I've tried to do that?" I say, talking and wiping my eyes at the same time. "For God's sake, Aliceanne, I'm *dying* . . . and it's not *my* fault."

"Of course it's not," says Aliceanne. "It's not your fault, and it's not their fault either. But the question still remains, what are you going to do now?"

"Well," I say, sniffling, "I guess I was hoping for just a little more help. I mean, is that so much to ask? After all the sacrifices I made? Like raising four children almost by myself, with my husband on the road the whole time. And managing my own illnesses too?" I choke up, the words lodging in my throat.

"Look," says Aliceanne. "I've just met someone who's perfect for you. He's a Boston-born Eastern healer by the name of Xavier Staub. Vietnam vet, sixth-degree black belt in Aikido, and he lives in Makaha. Get a pen and take down his number."

The next morning, I stare at the scrap of paper with Xavier's name and number on it. Makaha. All the way on the other side of the island. I put my hand on the phone, but don't pick it up.

Who am I kidding? It's too late for this. Just don't have the energy to drag myself around anymore.

No hope left.

As I packed our things into boxes for the move to North Carolina, I couldn't help thinking back to when Rob and I first moved in together. Not long before we were married. How we'd paused once we'd packed the moving van and looked at each other. Like we were both asking ourselves the same question. What in the hell are we doing?

Somehow, back then, we had convinced ourselves that it was just wedding jitters. We smiled at each other and shrugged it off. A little nervousness was only natural. Happened to everybody who made such a big decision.

Nine years later I had cold feet again, but for a different reason. I wasn't afraid of the commitment. I was afraid of the amount of traveling that came with Rob's new job.

So Rob left the NIH and he and I drove south, leaving the kids with his parents. The company put us up in a hotel and Rob and I started looking for a house. There was a lot to choose from since real estate prices in North Carolina were so much lower than they were in the D.C. area. I couldn't believe how much more space we'd have.

I don't think we were ever happier. Our new home was so much warmer than D.C. and I don't only mean the weather. I grew up just south of the Mason-Dixon line, but this new environment was really Southern living. People looked out for each other. Looked out for each other's children. And our next-door neighbors' twelve-year-old daughter was a built-in babysitter.

I remember our first years there as a time of giggles and haircuts and pulled teeth. Of traps made with wine boxes and string used to catch feral cats. Rabbits and hamsters and kittens and dogs. Scraped knees and cuts and bruises. Kisses and laughter and tears. Packs of kids running up and down the street.

It was everything I ever wanted. Except a husband who slept at home. True, there were no more calls from loan companies because we'd missed another car payment. But it was in North Carolina that I started to pass my nights in a bed far too big for just one person.

I don't know if it made me feel better or worse that Rob was out in the world saving lives. Only two years after we'd moved south the AIDS virus had become the leading cause of death for Americans between the ages of twenty-five and forty-four. And Rob's work was focused on developing drugs and drug therapies for the virus. Which meant he had to travel around the world continually, to visit the places where he had patients in clinical trials, and to keep up with his colleagues and new developments in the treatment of the disease.

That's when my health really started to decline. I'd never fully recovered from my pregnancies, and before I knew it I found myself in a whole new place, on my own with four young children. I was lonely and exhausted, and sleeping badly. I felt awful all the time.

Rob told me he thought I should see a psychiatrist. "Your problems aren't physiological," he'd say. "They're psychological."

We'd been having this conversation for years already. I'd tell Rob that I didn't feel well, and he'd tell me my problems were psychological, not physical. And he was the doctor, wasn't he? So, when Rob was still working for the NIH, I gave in and started seeing a psychologist. But because I was so thin, Dr. G. kept looking for an eating disorder, not signs of emotional distress.

And the same sort of thing happened when I started seeing another psychologist, Dr. H., in North Carolina. I wanted to talk to him about how I felt. But we never got around to that. Never even touched on any of the things I thought we'd talk about. Like feelings of abandonment. Or my suspicions that Rob was taking advantage of his travel schedule to cheat on me. I don't know. Maybe I thought it would sound selfish since we both knew my husband was doing work that was very important.

Instead we talked more and more about how Cat's birth had somehow jarred loose some long lost or deeply repressed memories of my childhood. And we talked about my recurring nightmares.

I'd been having them for years, but in North Carolina they began to come more and more often. Night after night I'd see the blue wallpaper in the spare bedroom in my grandmother's house. The room where my cousin, who stayed with my mother's mother over the summer, always touched me. I was only seven years old at the time. Only seven when I first felt the press of his tongue against my teeth. Felt his fingers trailing up my stomach, finding my chest. My nipples.

He wasn't the only one. Other nights I'd awaken with the smell of Father John's musty office at the summer camp in my nostrils. And then, like I was watching the feed from a hidden camera, I'd see the priest's head between my thirteen-year-old thighs. And it wasn't just me. By the end of that summer I could recognize the blank stares of all the girls he'd invited to his office for counseling.

And then I'd awaken and realize where I was. In North Carolina, in my home. Instinctively, I reached over to the other side of the bed for my husband. But more and more often my fingers found his pillow, untouched by his head.

In a panic, I'd jump out of bed. Rush into the nursery to hear the soft, steady rhythm of Cat's breathing. And then I'd lean into her crib, place my ear to her chest, and will my heart to beat in time with hers.

And then start counting the hours until Rob would be home again.

Chapter Sixteen

I WALK PAST THAT piece of paper with the name of Aliceanne's colleague on it every morning. Glance at the phone number. But I don't call. Instead I sign up for an art class. Something to keep me busy. And I buy myself a miniature Pinscher too because I'm sick of being alone all day.

I name the little dog "Be," as a reminder to myself to "be" in the moment. Not thinking of "to *be* or not to *be*," because that wasn't the question. At least not on good days. But no matter if it's a good day or a bad day, I keep just walking past that scrap of paper.

Xavier.

What kind of a name is that for an Eastern healer?

After I'd been seeing Dr. H. for six months or so, I could no longer hide the source of my nightmares from Rob. Whenever he was home, that is. So I finally told him about how my cousin would drag me upstairs into that little bedroom with the light blue wallpaper whenever Grandma was busy and how he ran his hands all over me and tried to put them in me. I told Rob about the priest too. He was furious. Said he'd beat the shit out of Father John if he could find him.

He never did. But I still loved him for saying it.

Finally talking to Rob took a great weight off my shoulders, because as the memories of abuse I'd suffered as a child started to leak out in therapy I'd been more and more afraid to tell him. What if he stopped loving me when he found out how damaged I was? Realized what a colossal mistake he'd made in marrying me? In having children with me? He'd leave us for sure once he knew. Wouldn't he?

The phone rings, startling me, and for one crazy moment I think it's Xavier calling me. But it can't be. Why would he? And how could he? As far as I know, he doesn't even have my number. Doesn't even know who I am.

"Hello."

It's Ada, our housekeeper in California. The conversation quickly turns surreal. The miniature pony Rob bought Cat when she was a kid is dead. They found her in her paddock that morning. And Rob's traveling, of course. And Ada's afraid to call Cat's cell.

No end to the sadness, it seems. I try to calm her down. Thank her for calling. Tell her I'll reach out to Cat. Then put the phone back in the cradle, glancing at Xavier's number again as I do. And then I close my eyes and remind myself that I have to keep breathing.

As the years went by in North Carolina, and the kids started to grow up, Rob was gone more and more often. Saving lives and offering hope to those who, just a few years earlier, had had none. Back when AIDS was still a death sentence.

And me? By then I was no longer a practicing RN, even if I had kept my license. I was a full-time mother. And just as importantly, a perfect wife.

Or at least that's what I tried to be. Always polishing my husband's image during his long absences. Which was the only way our neighbors ever got to know him. I mean, they knew who he was and what he did, but he was gone far too often to be part of the neighborhood. And when he did come home for a day or two, every now and then, we could never just have a simple meal together. He always wanted to go out to the best restaurant. Or better still, throw a big dinner party. With the

58

clean-up left until the next day. When he was back at work and the boys were in school.

I wonder if that's when Cat began to believe that being a woman meant taking care of the men and boys around you?

Other times, when Rob was home, he'd get all the kids in the car and go someplace fun. He'd even take the neighbors' kids. And pay for everything. But he was never around when it was time to call the plumber. Or to check the kids' homework. Or to meet their teachers. Or to kick a soccer ball around or throw a baseball. Or to make sure the kids were all in bed when they were supposed to be.

Chapter Seventeen

I<small>T'S A TYPICALLY</small> warm Hawaiian morning in late September. I check my blood sugar and blood pressure. No change. I totter out onto the deck, holding on to whatever's at hand until I reach a chair. Above me, in the trees, the tropical birds squawk at each other and flap their wings.

Once I've settled myself in the chair, my eyes go right to the water. As if I were a kid on a beach. I wonder if I'll ever get my feet wet again.

Music's coming from somewhere nearby, but I can't make out the tune at first. That song from *Dirty Dancing*, maybe?

I didn't know it then of course, but the summer of 1992 was probably the high point of my young married life. With four young children to take care of, I guess I was too busy to notice, but with Rob on the road all the time I had to do everything. Keep the house clean. Pay the bills. Do the shopping. Cook the meals. Wash the clothes. Cut the grass. And try not to wonder if my husband was fooling around when he was out of town.

I'd never been blind to the way women looked at him. Talked to him. Touched him. Besides, he told me about it himself. Many times. Drinking loosened his tongue, and like everyone in his family he loved to drink. And when he did, he'd tell me about all the women coming on to him. And then the next day he'd look at me like I was crazy and say

I'd imagined it. But I hadn't. And now I wonder if he was gas-lighting me all the way back then. Telling me something and then denying everything. Making me doubt my own memory.

But if my memory was unreliable, it had nothing to do with alcohol. I quit drinking when I got pregnant with Liam.

Then there was the black onyx necklace he gave me after a trip to New York. Just because, he'd said. Because he'd seen it and thought I'd like it.

And there was my birthday in the late summer of 1994. As it happened Rob's younger brother, Tom, had the same birthday I did, and he had joined us to celebrate in North Carolina. Afterward, once the kids were in bed, Rob talked him into going out to a strip club.

"Come on, it'll be fun," said Rob. "It's your birthday. You need to go out and do something crazy."

Seemed like Rob needed to get out and do something crazy too.

Chapter Eighteen

E VERY NOW AND then, as the warm autumn days go by in the white house on Oahu, it occurs to me that perhaps I'm not meant to die. But if I don't, what am I going to do? Go back to California? That isn't going to change anything. My doctors have already done everything they can for me. Or to me.

I try to remember when it was that Rob called me from San Francisco. The year 1995? No. Cat was two. So it was 1996.

"You won't believe how blue the skies are out here, sweetie," Rob told me over the phone.

He had taken a job at another pharmaceutical company. Without even mentioning it to me. And since this company's headquarters were in Silicon Valley, it was time to pack everything up again. And this time there was a lot more to pack up. To say nothing of some of the things we couldn't pack and would have to leave behind. Like the big comfortable house. And the neighbors who had become family. And the gentle, dependable rhythm of life in North Carolina.

He understood, Rob said. He really did. But he'd taken the job in California because he could continue his work and make even more money. No one in the family could be against that. Even if it did mean traveling a little more.

"Hey, look at the bright side," he said. "At least the kids are a little older this time."

They were. Almost four years older. Old enough to know what was going on. Old enough to know that they loved living in North Carolina and didn't want to move. And to know that I didn't want to move either.

A few months later we were settled in a smaller but much more expensive house. In a wealthy and competitive suburb of Silicon Valley. And it was there that our family really began to veer off track and our kids started getting into trouble.

We had moved from a big sunny house in a family-friendly neighborhood to a tight dark space in one of the most expensive real estate markets in the country. And this new neighborhood had the bratty kids and status-conscious moms and driven-to-succeed husbands that went with it.

But I didn't know that yet. All I knew was that our new house cost more than five times what we got for our first house. And even though I'd left the farm and had never looked back, I couldn't help thinking how many acres of farmland we could have bought with that kind of money.

But money, according to Rob, was no longer an issue. And it never would be again, to hear him tell it. The new company had even given him a bridge loan for a down payment on the house. And between his salary and stock options, neither one of us would be pulling night shifts in an ER ever again. Or opening walk-in clinics to make sure we could cover the car payment. We were finally living the dream.

So, where were all the night sweats coming from?

Chapter Nineteen

NGRY AND ALONE, I give up waiting by the phone and trudge through the sand just south of Kaneohe Bay. Alone, that is, if you don't count Beatrice. The little dog's name is growing almost as fast as she is.

During the time we lived in Northern California, I don't have a single memory of feeling physically well. What I do remember is feeling lonely. And overwhelmed. And more and more guilty as all of our kids eventually found their way into trouble.

Finally, I convinced Rob that Liam ought to talk to someone. Maybe a psychologist. Before long, Dr. S. was working with our entire family, separately and together. Including Rob, when his schedule would allow it. Which wasn't very often.

Rob continued to press me to see a psychiatrist. "But I'm already seeing someone," I'd respond.

And then another round of lab tests my internist had ordered came back normal.

"Admit it, Jules, there's nothing wrong with you," said Rob, holding out a sheaf of papers. "The labs don't lie. They're all within normal ranges. Which means you need to find another...."

"... another what? Another psychologist?"

"No. Not another psychologist. They can't prescribe meds."

When I didn't respond, he went on. "I think you should see a psychiatrist. So he can prescribe meds."

Which wasn't that surprising. What else would an M.D. employed by Big Pharma think a patient needed, if all the labs kept coming in normal? Which obviously meant my symptoms had to be a manifestation of some sort of psychological disorder.

In other words, I was crazy.

So I started seeing Dr. Y., and he began prescribing a series of antidepressants. First Trazodone. Then Ativan. Finally, Buspar. I took the meds like a good girl, but in my heart I still knew that something else was wrong with me. Something at my core.

I was a registered nurse after all, and a mother too, and I believed that patients intuitively knew when something was wrong with them.

The question was, would anyone listen?

The white sand glitters. The turquoise waters of the Pacific sparkle in the sunlight. My little dog Beatrice is off the leash and running free. But I can't keep up with her. Not with my left foot still in a walking cast.

Can it really be that almost thirty years have gone by since Rob and I met? Has it really been more than fourteen years since we moved to the west coast?

I've been sick for so long I can't even imagine anymore what it feels like to be well. For years now, I've been getting up every morning and dressing in my illnesses. And as uncomfortable as they are, they're all I know. All I've got in the emotional closet.

If I ever got well, I wouldn't have anything to wear.

As my physical and mental condition worsened, my husband began to look at me as if I were a stranger.

"You can't blame me for this," Rob said. "You were broken when I met you."

I swallowed that casual cruelty the same way I continued to swallow *the antidepressants, without much hope that things would get better. And Rob, who never stopped moving, was more and more annoyed by my failure to keep up. Not that anyone else could have. By that time in our life he was living on the road. Singapore. Australia. Munich. He had important work to do. And while he saved lives, we spent the money he made.*

"I'm tired," I told him over the phone. "I just can't do this anymore."

"Yes, you can," he said. "And don't forget to call the caterer about the dinner party on Tuesday."

It felt like everything was falling apart. Our children kept getting in trouble. One morning, Liam drove his car off the road and down a steep incline not a mile from the house. Later that same day, Nathan had an accident too.

But the dinner party was a huge success.

Chapter Twenty

ON OAHU, I eat by myself. Don't cook much. Somedays it seems like I get by on nothing more than cigarettes and diet soda. And my meds of course.

A quick trip into town becomes a major expedition. Takes me an hour just to get ready. To be sure I've got everything I need. Injectable steroids are at the top of the list. If somebody runs a red light and hits me, my body won't be able to provide enough adrenaline to get me out of the car.

Steroids. Check. Insulin. Check. Pump. Check.

A few nights after the dinner party, Rob and I went out to dinner.

"What's wrong?" he asked me.

I shrugged.

"I think the antidepressants are messing with my head. I can't think anymore."

He stared at me without saying a word.

"I'm not crazy," I said, looking back at him from across the table. "Something is really and truly wrong with me."

He drew in a deep breath and shook his head. "You've got the best doctors at Stanford," he said, "and your labs are normal. Sooner or later you've just got to trust me. And trust your medical team. If there were something wrong with you, we'd know."

He reached across the table and put his hand on mine. "It's all in your head," he said.

I started to cry. Which Rob hated. Especially when we were in public.

"I'm telling you, something is wrong with me," I said again, tears streaming down my cheeks. "You have to believe me."

He went back to eating his dinner. "Don't get hysterical," he said, between bites.

I just picked at my food. Tired and desperate, I just wanted to go home. But I wasn't going to give in. Again.

"If there's nothing wrong with me, why do I get a fever every single night?" I asked him. "Explain that to me. Why do I get a fever, every single night, right around seven?"

Rob looked up. Then put his knife and fork down. "What'd you say?"

Finally, I had his attention.

"I said, I get a fever every night around seven o'clock. That's got to mean something?"

He sat back in his chair and looked at me like I was a new patient. "Sounds like a circadian rhythm," he said, more to himself than to me. Then he waved the waiter over, paid our bill and took me home.

"I have some reading to do," he said. I nodded, then dragged myself upstairs and fell asleep.

He woke me up in the wee hours of the morning. "We have to go to the hospital immediately."

When we got there, a nurse drew a vial of blood. And this time my lab work didn't come back normal. My cortisol levels were dangerously low. They were so low, in fact, that even a small crisis might have put me in a coma. Finally, I had a name for what I'd been feeling.

Addison's disease. My adrenal system had almost shut down. But at least I finally had a diagnosis.

Better sick than crazy.

I continue to look at the scrap of paper with Xavier's number on it. Every morning. It's right there on the counter next to the tea kettle on the stove. Some days I even pick it up and trail a finger across the ink scrawl. Like a blind person reading Braille.

I don't have the strength to try again. My hopes have been dashed too many times.

But waiting is driving me out of my mind. I pick up the phone and call the number. The phone rings three times.

"This is Xavier." He's from Boston all right. And he hasn't lost his accent.

I make an appointment for the following Tuesday.

Part III
Hoping

Chapter Twenty-One

"**D**on't get too excited, Mom," says Liam as he drives up the western shore of Oahu. We're heading toward Makaha, a blue-collar town on the northwestern corner of the island. About an hour's drive from Kaneohe Bay.

I don't respond to his warning. Just pat him on the knee and look out his open window at the eternal ocean, stretching away to the west.

After months of inaction I feel the old thrill of hope. But I also sense that Liam is, as usual, wondering what this latest scheme will mean to him. And after all the times he's seen me get my hopes up, only to see me deteriorate even further, I can understand his apprehension. None of them allow themselves to hope anymore. Not even Rob, despite his medical degree. And some days I feel the same way.

But deep inside me, where no one else can hear it, hope still whispers.

"This time it's really going to work. This time you're going to show them all and get well."

As Liam pulls up, Xavier stands at the end of his gravel driveway. He's wearing a faded blue t-shirt and a pair of gray sweatpants. He's thin, but clearly in good shape. Rumpled gray hair, like he's just walked through a wind tunnel. An honest smile on his face, framed by a Fu Manchu mustache beneath a slightly hooked nose.

And if Aliceanne is right, this ex-biker-looking martial artist turned Eastern healer is just the guy I've been looking for.

And then his eyes catch mine. They're glacier-blue, and they pierce mine like lasers. Like he's scanning me. Searching beneath the steroid-induced swelling. Looking past the scars of my twelve surgeries. Trying to see the woman I used to be. Or the woman I could be. And I can't help wondering if the woman he sees is worth saving.

Inside, Xavier settles himself on the edge of the treatment table and folds his hands in his lap. I'm a little uncomfortable, so I wait for him to begin the intake process. You know, to ask me about my medical history. I mean, even though he's a practitioner of traditional Chinese medicine and not an MD, he'll still need *some* background information, won't he?

But he doesn't ask me any of the usual questions. In fact, he doesn't ask me anything at all. He just sits there and stares at me.

"You're an abused woman," he says finally, without a preamble.

The words almost knock the wind out of me. "An abused woman? I am not."

Ridiculous. Absurd.

"Yes," he says again, "you are."

I shake my head, offended. What does Aliceanne see in this guy anyway?

"I'm not an abused woman," I say, having trouble getting the words out. He's wrong. Abused women hide in dark rooms. Wipe away tears with trembling hands. Use makeup to cover unexplainable bruises. Abused women cower and make themselves small. So they're harder to hit.

I just don't fit that description.

I'm married to a leading research physician, a man who has never and would never lay a hand on me in anger. I am the mother of four beautiful children just beginning their lives as young adults. I have some great friends. Women I love and trust and respect. I whip up dinner parties that our guests talk about for weeks afterward. I live in one of the most beautiful and exclusive places in the country. And vacation in the paradise that is Hawaii. How can this guy call me an abused woman?

Okay, I'm sick. And probably dying. But not abused.

Xavier just sits there and looks at me. Like he too can hear the voice in my head talking away. If he wanted to. But he's in no particular rush. Willing to wait until I quit trying to fool myself.

"How many surgeries have you had?" he asks, as if he already knows, but wants to hear it from me. And dutiful patient that I am, I take a deep breath and start ticking them off. Like I'm reading from a grocery list, one that I've read out loud, over and over again. As the list got longer and longer.

A tonsillectomy when I was three. Removal of a melanoma on my chest at seventeen. Surgery for an arthritic nodule on my right wrist at nineteen. An inguinal hernia repaired once during my second pregnancy, and then again right after Nathan was born. Cataract surgery. Stomach fundoplication. Four sinus surgeries including one that took six hours. Removal of my gallbladder.

"Is that all?"

"No," I say, eager to show him just how wrong he is. "That's just the surgeries. I've had two GI bleeds, one of which required a blood transfusion. Three episodes of kidney stones. Asthma. Bronchiectasis. Chronic arthritis. Plus a fever of unknown origin that kept me in the hospital for three weeks. I can't even remember how many bone marrow biopsies they took for that one. And then there was the fever that left me in a coma for a day and a half when Cat and I were visiting Sherry and her family in North Carolina."

I sit up a little straighter, as if I've just presented my resume.

Xavier keeps his eyes on mine.

"So, you've had all those surgeries, and you still say you're not an abused woman."

What he's saying begins to sink in.

"The human body," he says, "isn't meant to be cut into that many times."

He steps out of the treatment room so I can change into a Bird-of-Paradise sarong. I slip out of my shirt and my bra and tie the sarong around my neck so my chest is covered and my back exposed. Then I climb onto the treatment table, worried that it may not support all two hundred pounds of me.

Without a word Xavier comes back into the room and begins to knead the flesh along my spine. He doesn't seem to be in any sort of a hurry. "Try to relax into the table."

Is he kidding?

"Just try to release your mind," he goes on. "Let go of your thoughts."

I do my best to relax as he works the muscles of my thighs, shoulders and calves, but I stiffen the moment I feel acupuncture needles prick the tops of my feet and the insides of my wrists.

"Don't tense up," he tells me. "Just relax, and let the needles unblock the energies along your meridians."

It's not the first time I've had acupuncture. But it's the first time from someone who's called me an abused woman. And thinking about that makes it impossible for me to relax. My thoughts scatter. I panic.

Abused? It can't be true, can it?

And yet fifteen minutes later, as I lie on my back with an aromatic sachet resting on my eyes and a cool island breeze blowing gently over my skin, some part of me already knows that he's right.

Which means everyone else was wrong all these years.

Including my doctors.

And me.

Chapter Twenty-Two

ACK IN THE year 2000, on the night that follow-up tests confirmed Rob's diagnosis of Addison's disease, I briefly became an overnight medical celebrity. After all, in America only one out of every hundred thousand people suffers from the disease. Most doctors never even see a single case. So, once they admitted me, Rob strutted around the hospital like a peacock. And when the other doctors and nurses found out, everybody patted him on the back like he was a new father or something.

I know it sounds crazy, but when the doctor told me I was sick it made me happy. Really happy. This was what I'd been praying for. Finally something in the blood work.

For years, I'd been saying something was physically wrong with me. And for years I'd asked for help. Or at the very least a little understanding. Someone who believed me. Who believed that I was telling the truth. That it wasn't all in my head.

What had I gotten instead? Antidepressants.

But not that night. When the doctor saw the level of cortisol in my plasma everything changed. Within an hour I had traded in my Trazodone for the steroid Prednisone.

I still have my early lab reports. That is, the ones that came immediately after my diagnosis. And of course the hundreds and hundreds of lab reports that came afterward. They'd probably be pretty confusing to most people. But as a nurse I'd been reading them for years. I knew just what to look for and where to find it, how to keep an eye on meaningful changes. They were almost like horoscopes, changing every day depending on the alignment of the stars. And now my stars had finally lined up.

And lab reports don't just show test results. They also show reference ranges for the values being tested. In the case of the hormone cortisol, these ranges change over the course of the day. From 8:00 to 10:00 AM they generally fall between 4 – 25 MCG/DL. That stands for micrograms per deciliter. And then from 4:00 to 6:00 PM they usually fall between 2 – 12 MCG/DL.

In the morning of March 8, 2000, my cortisol plasma level was 0.8. Which meant that Rob's timely diagnosis was little short of a miracle. Put another way, there were numerous circumstances under which I might have died. A routine car crash could have done it.

And Rob was the one who had saved me. Again. First he'd shown me a way out of the Maryland farmland. Then we brought four children into the world together. We had worked our way out of the middle class. And now he'd saved my life by seeing, as no one else had, that I suffered from an extremely rare disease.

Addison's disease is a rare chronic endocrine disorder characterized by low functioning adrenal glands. Or in my case, non-functioning adrenal glands. They're triangle-shaped and look like little elves' caps perched on top of the kidneys. And they produce hormones like cortisol and adrenaline, which maintain a homeostatic environment in the body. Which means they keep things in balance over time.

With Addison's, the adrenals can't make sufficient amounts of cortisol. And cortisol is one of the primary fight-or-flight hormones. It does several things for the body. During times of stress, it increases sugars in the bloodstream and it enhances the use of those sugars in the brain. It also governs the substances the body uses to repair tissue. And during times of fight-or-flight it also slows non-essential functions of the body, like digestion, reproduction and growth. If a car is about to hit you, your body no longer cares about your stomach. It just wants you to be able to contract and expand the muscles in your arms and legs.

80

But cortisol levels aren't constant. They fluctuate according to a circadian rhythm, continually rising and falling in response to the earth's cycle of light and dark. Unfortunately, synthetic steroids like Prednisone don't perfectly mimic the natural cycle of the adrenal glands. The best they can do is approximate them. So I had to wear an emergency alert bracelet and carry injectable steroids with me at all times. The thing is that at the time, there was no way to quickly and reliably measure cortisol levels. If my body were challenged by a car accident, for instance, I could go into shock and die without an immediate steroid injection.

But there's something else that's even worse. Addison's is an autoimmune disease. It means that your white blood cells incorrectly identify your *own* healthy cells as foreign bodies. And then they attack them. As if they were splinters. Or cancer cells.

So *that* was what was wrong with me. I was attacking myself from the inside.

Chapter Twenty-Three

I RETURN TO MAKAHA for my second appointment with Xavier. Again, I change out of my clothes and lie down on his treatment table, wearing nothing more than a light blue sarong.

It is the late fall of 2010. I am forty-nine years old. I weigh almost two hundred pounds. I have a hump on my back from the steroids. My skin is like paper. My arms and legs are like sticks. My doctors use the word *cushingoid* to describe what I look like. But do yourself a favor. Don't look it up. You don't want an image of a naked cushingoid woman in your head. And neither do I. Which is why I avoid mirrors.

When I make the appointment for the session, Xavier encourages me to drive across the island myself. "You've got to stop depending on others. Take control of your own healing."

Take control of my own healing? Is he kidding? That's *exactly* what I've been doing for the last ten years. Managing the team of doctors who managed my care.

Besides, it's a bit of a trek from Kaneohe Bay to Xavier's compound in Makaha. And Liam isn't happy about me driving there on my own. "I don't care if he told you to . . ."

". . . he didn't *tell* me to. He just suggested it."

Liam stares at me, almost like his father does. "Well, what if your blood sugar drops while you're driving?"

Liam doesn't like the neighborhood either. He's worried I might get mugged. But I'm not worried. No one even notices a woman who looks like I do. Not now. I'm overweight, weirdly puffy, and not wearing any tell-tale fancy jewelry or clothes. Children might stare at me, but adults look away. No mugger's going to take a second look.

Besides, I'm going to be driving our old pickup truck, which is about the only thing around here that's as beat up as I am. So no worries about another scratch or a dent. And it's not like I'm driving through some gritty inner-city slum. The whole island of Oahu is about as close as you can get to heaven on earth. The breeze is warm and playful. White clouds drift across the light blue sky. As the truck rumbles north up the coast the lush green forests of the Ko`olau mountains loom to my right. The Pacific glitters calmly on my left, living up to its name.

"Let's start with three treatments a week," says Xavier. I'm stretched out face down on the table. "We need to get your Qi moving again."

"My Qi?" I say, although I already know what Qi is. Or at least I think I do. But I want to know what *he* thinks it is.

"Your Qi is your life force," says Xavier, as he massages my lower spine. "Chinese medicine teaches us that we have twelve major meridians. If it helps, you can think of them as energy pathways, running through our bodies. And when our Qi flows freely through our meridians, we're healthy."

So that's the problem. I've got Qi that doesn't flow. Like a shower backing up when the drain is clogged with hair. Except I've got hairballs in my *meridians*.

Chapter Twenty-Four

As I wore my freshly-diagnosed Addison's disease like a glittering tiara, physicians at the teaching hospital stopped to see me as they and their interns made their morning rounds. And who doesn't like a little attention? Especially after years of listening to my doctors tell me that there was nothing physically wrong with me. Now that everybody knew better, I'd sit there dutifully on an exam table while the interns and residents poked and prodded and questioned me, and then swept out of the room like a pack of horses following their stallion.

Unless Rob accompanied me. Whenever he took me to my appointments the doctors acted as if I weren't even there. They talked only to him. As if I were incapable of communicating or understanding. Even though I was an RN, I had become nothing more than an interesting case. No longer a person but a condition to be treated.

Never a patient, who might one day heal.

Xavier's treatment room is nothing like any hospital I've ever been in. Still, I feel like a patient anesthetized for surgery whenever I lie down on his table. I know it's the wrong mental image. But after years and years of treatments and medications and surgeries, that's just the way I think. You get well in doctors' offices and hospitals. You monitor your blood and take drugs.

Lots and lots of drugs.

Xavier places another aromatic sachet over my eyes and then moves around me, acupuncture needles in hand. But I'm not really feeling any better. Instead, I'm starting to feel like a pincushion. And I can't help wondering exactly how long this process is supposed to take.

A month?

Six months?

A year, God forbid?

"You know, it's okay if you die," Xavier says, slipping another needle into me.

It's a little like somebody telling you you've got cancer, while you're being fitted for a dress. It comes from so far out of nowhere, I can't process what he's saying. And when I do finally get it, I don't know what to say. I mean, aren't those about the last words you want to hear out of your healer's mouth? Kind of defeats the whole purpose of healing doesn't it? And it's not much of a business model either. Eliminates the whole repeat customer thing. No testimonials either.

"What did you say?" I ask, still in the dark, the lightly scented sachet covering my eyes.

"I said, it's okay if you die. In fact, you can drop dead this second, and nobody'll care."

Wait a minute. Haven't I heard this before? From Aliceanne, maybe? Yeah. You have permission to die. That's what she'd said. I'd almost forgotten. Like that's what I'd been waiting for. Okay, in a way it *was* what I'd been waiting for. But I never told *her* that.

No wonder she thinks this guy's the one for me.

I'll tell you one thing, I can't even *imagine* my doctors in California telling me it's okay for me to die. To them, death means failure. Death means defeat. And accepting it without a battle isn't an option. To them, this would be the height of medical irresponsibility. If a hospital were a church, the idea would be blasphemous.

Let's schedule another CAT scan, they'd say. Or, we need another biopsy. Or, when was her last CBC? Maybe we should try another medication.

86

But unlike Aliceanne, Xavier isn't giving me *permission* to die. He's telling me *it doesn't matter if I die.*

And as that thought darts through my mind, like a bird caught indoors looking for a way out, Xavier starts to remove the acupuncture needles. I fume under the sachet, which is almost *too* fragrant now. Like it's going to make me sick. And all I can hear is Xavier's slow, rhythmic breathing.

"Your kids don't give a shit about you," he says, "and neither does your husband."

He then removes the sachet and rocks me up into a sitting position at the edge of the treatment table. I squint in the harsh afternoon sunlight, my eyes adjusting slowly, and he leaves me there as he disposes of the used acupuncture needles.

I'm an abused woman.

It doesn't matter if I die.

No one cares.

Did he really just say those things to me? Does he really mean them? Maybe my insulin's off. Or my steroids are low. Or maybe I'm a little light-headed because I haven't had enough to eat.

I want to disagree with what he's said. And I want to hate him for saying it. But I don't and I can't because I know he's at least a little right. And what I begin to feel as I think it over, oddly enough, is relief. No one has spoken to me with that sort of merciless honesty. Not for years. My doctors have all coddled me, like I'm a sick child who can't understand what's going on. With the exception of my endocrinologist, maybe. But even she's never slapped me across the face, metaphorically speaking, quite like that. I'm talking about the kind of open-handed slap that's meant to snap you out of something.

But it still stings.

Chapter Twenty-Five

I N THE SPRING of 2000, a couple weeks after they started giving me Prednisone to treat the Addison's diagnosis, my family practitioner sent me to see an endocrinologist for further tests. Her first report is below.

Thank you for the opportunity to evaluate Julie R., a 38-year-old married. R.N., who has recently received a diagnosis of primary adrenal insufficiency.

HPI: The patient reports that she has had problems with nausea and poor appetite for at least a year or more. Her weight is relatively stable at 120 pounds but she has weighed as little as 100 pounds. When she does eat she tends to feel worse, especially if she eats red meat. She has noted tachycardia, and often feels weak, shaky and lightheaded. She has noted problems with concentration and memory for several months. Her skin has recently become darker, particularly over recent scars and especially around her eyes. Blood pressure 110/70. Pulse 110. No postural changes reported. She has tried eating a large quantity of salt and notes that this makes her feel better.

The patient was started by her physician husband on Prednisone 5 mg. in the evening and felt improved within a few hours. Presently she is taking Prednisone 10 mg. a.m. and 5 mg. mid-afternoon.

The patient has had considerable workup prior to her visit here today. She had a CT of her chest, abdomen and pelvis which showed bilateral ovarian vein thromboses of unknown significance. There were no unusual findings in the chest. Her sed rate was normal.

Other problems noted by the patient include irregular menses for several years. More recently they occur every 4-8 weeks. She has had night sweats for 15 years off and on. They seem to be somewhat improved on Prednisone. Chest X-ray and PPD have been negative in the past. She has had considerable GI workup for nausea and diarrhea and H. pylori test was reportedly negative. Recently she has been found to be anemic, but this may be due to medication (Dapsone). In fact her recent hemoglobin has risen from 10 to 12.3.

Even then, long before my list of medications lengthened, the drugs I was taking had begun to cause problems of their own. But that's the great thing about Western medicine. There's always something else to take for that.

MEDICATIONS: Prednisone 10 mg. q a.m., 5 mg. q mid-afternoon.

ALLERGIES: Tagamet – gastroparesis. Dapsone – hemolytic anemia. Sulfa – swelling.

HCATTS: Occasional smoking. Caffeine none. Alcohol minimal.

The report was dated March 24, 2000 and was sent to my internist. No one else was copied.

Liam turned sixteen about a week after my initial consultation with the endocrinologist. He remembers that period as the beginning of my "chronic" illness. That is when I started making daily trips to one doctor or another, as opposed to the weekly visits I had been making after we moved west. He also points to this as the beginning of my physical problems, as opposed to the emotional issues I had in North Carolina. The place he was happiest as a child.

Which just goes to show that you can't hide anything from your kids, no matter how hard you try. It also meant that Rob and I had already failed our children, just like my parents had failed me. But there was no turning the clock back. With the Addison's diagnosis I had no choice but to take care of myself, or I'd never be able to take care of any of them again.

Chapter Twenty-Six

"WHAT IF NONE of it's true?"

I'm lying on Xavier's treatment table half asleep. The question comes out of nowhere.

"What if none of *what* is true?" I say.

"What if none of what your doctors told you is true?" Xavier asks me again, continuing to massage my body. "What if your illnesses are just an illusion? One that you and your doctors created?"

"My doctors and I didn't *create* anything," I say, getting up on my elbows and turning my head to look back at him. "And I've got the labs to prove it."

"I'm sure you do," he says, gently guiding my head down to the mat and then going back to work on my lower back. "But that's not my point. What if your body doesn't *need* all the drugs you're taking?"

I can't believe what I'm hearing. Doesn't he understand how sick I am? "If I don't take my steroids," I say, shifting my weight until I'm comfortable on the table again, "I could fall into a coma and die."

"Could you?" he says, kneading the lower part of my spine. "How do you know?"

I get back up on my elbows. "I know because I'm a registered nurse. Plus my husband's a physician, to say nothing of my doctors, who just happen to be the best doctors in the whole world."

"If you say so," he continues, the tension in my spine fading with the touch of his fingers. "But what if it's *not* true?"

Now I'm starting to get irritated. I almost say something, but at the last moment I take a deep breath and press my lips together again. Because now I get it. This is just part of the treatment. He's asking me questions to shake me up. To encourage me to look at my illnesses in a different way. To think about the possibility that there might be more than one way to heal. Pretty clever.

But that doesn't change the fact that my adult life has been built around my belief in Western medicine. My entire identity has really. I'm an RN. My husband is an M.D. And I'm alive today only because I was lucky enough to assemble a great medical team. People I've known and worked with for ten years now. Some of whom have become good friends. So for me to accept the idea that my body might *not* need all the medications I'm taking, or that my diagnoses are inaccurate is a lot to ask.

Honestly, it's never even occurred to me to question my husband's or my doctors' diagnoses. Why would I? I was sure *something* was wrong with me. I just didn't know what name to give it.

Besides, in the Western world, we endow our physicians with god-like powers. Why else would we wait in densely packed, poorly lit, uncomfortable rooms full of sick people until our doctors finally get around to seeing us? Who else would we sit still for as they tell us all about ourselves, even though they don't really know us and won't spend more than a half a day with us over the course of our entire lives? Who else but our doctors? And most of us do this without any real understanding of what our doctors are doing. Or more importantly *why* they're doing it.

But that wasn't the case with me.

I knew. And my husband knew what they were doing, too.

"So, you're saying they couldn't possibly be wrong?" Xavier asks quietly, working on one of my legs. "That the drugs couldn't possibly be making things worse, instead of better?"

Stubbornly refusing to concede the point, I say, "If it weren't for the meds I'd have died years ago."

"Oh," he says, as if he'd never thought of such a thing. "So, it's

94

simply *impossible* that they've been treating your symptoms, instead of the source of your illnesses?"

A deafening silence falls over the small room. I draw a deep breath in through my nose. "I guess it's *possible*," I say. "But blood tests don't lie. And mine say I've got Addison's disease, which means my adrenal glands aren't producing enough corticosteroids. And since Addison's can't be cured, what else can they do but give me synthetic steroids?"

He begins to work on my right leg, his fingers probing for tension. "*Your* doctors might call it Addison's disease," he says. "But as an Eastern healer, I would call it emotional malnutrition."

Chapter Twenty-Seven

IN THE FALL of 2000, six months after my Addison's diagnosis, my doctors in California determined that I suffered from Crohn's disease too. Now the new millennium had really kicked in.

Crohn's disease is a painful inflammatory bowel disease, and there's no known cure. But just the same, I felt like driving around the neighborhood and broadcasting the news from a loudspeaker. That is, the news that I'd really been sick, and for a long time.

Sick. Not crazy.

And the additional diagnosis meant there was no longer any doubt that what I'd been telling everyone for years was really true. My problems were physical. Not psychological.

Okay. Maybe they were a little of both. But at least they weren't *all* psychological. Besides who could possibly feel as badly as I did for so many years without some kind of psychological repercussions? It was only natural.

My doctors prescribed an IV infusion of Remicade, which was supposed to reduce inflammation, for the Crohn's. But almost immediately, I developed a fever of unknown origin. And since doctors hate a fever of unknown origin, that led to a series of bone marrow biopsies and spinal taps. Which revealed granulomatous lesions common with Crohn's. But unlike most patients with Crohn's, the lesions showed up in organs outside my bowel. And that led my doctors to reclassify my second major autoimmune disease as metastatic Crohn's.

Believe me, nothing good ever begins with the word "metastatic." When something metastasizes it spreads from its original site. Which is why most people associate the word with cancer because that's how most cancers spread. Like seeds from a tree, falling on moving water. Drifting downstream until they wash up on shore and take root and grow until they block the sunlight and drink the river dry. And you die.

So in addition to the Remicade, my doctors put me on the broad-spectrum antibiotic Levaquin for almost two years. Humira followed the Remicade. I had to give myself a weekly injection. Eight hundred dollars a pop if you didn't have the kind of insurance we did. And it hurt like hell.

Their hope was that the Humira would treat the Crohn's lesions in my bowel so I could better absorb the steroids for the Addison's. That way we could lower the number of steroids I was taking. Unfortunately, the Humira led to a series of infections—mostly sinus infections and kidney infections—which resulted in long hospital stays.

Which meant our kids now had two absentee parents.

That year, on the day before Thanksgiving, Liam was arrested for driving under the influence and possession. Two felonies and a misdemeanor. He was only sixteen years old.

Chapter Twenty-Eight

I'VE GOTTEN INTO the habit of paying Xavier as soon as I arrive for a treatment. Otherwise I'm halfway home before I remember. Guess I've gotten too used to having the best healthcare money can buy. And to being utterly in the dark about what it all costs. Doctor's visits and consults. Treatments, medications, wheelchairs and surgeries. I mean, over ten years the medications alone probably added up to more than a million dollars. But we never got a single bill. Just an invoice for all the copays at the end of the month. Which Rob would pay. The insurance covered everything else.

A session of acupuncture and massage at the Makaha Wellness Center cost seventy dollars an hour. I could easily spend twice that on a pair of shoes. And I know Rob pays more than that for the *least* expensive bottle in his wine cellar.

Sometimes, if Xavier does something else in addition to the acupuncture and massage, the cost is a little bit more. Like moxa, which involves burning dried, ground mugwort on certain parts of the body. Don't ask me why. But it's also true that if you can't pay, he treats you just the same. I've seen it happen all the time. And the same goes for Louise, his partner. There's no charge for their twice-weekly Aikido sessions. They ask only for donations from those who can afford them.

After our session one day, Xavier leaves me alone in the treatment room while I put my clothes back on.

"Disease is not natural," he says when he walks back into the room. "It's a signal that something is wrong. That you are not connected with essence . . ."

". . . which is what, exactly?"

"The source of all energy . . . of all that is."

He looks into my eyes, trying to see if I've heard and understood what he's saying.

"I get it," I respond. "Disease isn't natural."

His eyes stay on mine a moment longer. "Our spirits come into this world innocent and whole," he says, tilting his head to steer me toward the door. "But they don't stay that way for long. Before we can learn who we really are, our parents, our society, our schools and our churches all try to convince us that we were born in sin. That we are not innocent, but *guilty* at birth. That we are not naturally *whole*. That we must *earn* God's love."

He doesn't know it, but he's preaching to the choir. I learned that I had to earn love at a very young age.

"But it's not true," he continues. "We *are* born whole. *You* were born whole. But somewhere along the way, you were separated from essence. And as strange as it must sound, your diseases are now your beacons. They'll guide you back to your birthright, and to wholeness, if you allow them to."

We walk down his gravel driveway toward the truck. I'm trying to make sense of everything Xavier's just told me, but he doesn't give me enough time. He just keeps going. "We're all just drops of water in a vast and infinite ocean."

Heard that one before.

"But that doesn't mean we're alone," he continues. "Or insignificant. It means only that we are all part of something greater than ourselves. That we are all connected to each other. To everything. To essence."

I'm still trying to catch up with that bit about no longer being whole. I'd always thought my illnesses were somehow connected to the feeling of emptiness I had from the time I was a child. But I'm almost fifty now. And after so much time has gone by, how in the hell am I going to fill that empty space? Acupuncture and massage

100

aren't going to do it. And neither is therapy. I've been in and out of psychologists' and psychiatrists' offices for nearly twenty years.

Xavier's voice comes through my thoughts.

"If you're willing to work, I think I can help you heal."

None of my doctors ever said *anything* like that to me. They just talked about managing my diseases. Not curing them. And about managing the side effects of all the meds I take. "You really think I can get well?"

He looks into my eyes again and nods. "If you're willing to make some changes. And to let me teach you how to get out of your own way."

I have no idea what he means. And if I weren't so tired I would ask to read the fine print before agreeing to give what he's suggesting a try. But I don't.

Chapter Twenty-Nine

I KNOW I MUST sound like a typical Silicon Valley mom, but Liam really didn't deserve to get arrested on the night before Thanksgiving. It wasn't his fault. Okay, maybe it was. But he didn't go looking for it.

I'll never forget that day. November 23rd, 2000. This was just a few months after my Crohn's diagnosis. He'd been hanging out with one of his friends, and this friend had an older brother who was in Palo Alto, and he needed a ride home. So Liam drove his friend down the hill into town.

The problem was the older brother was drunk when they got there and started arguing with one of his friends right on the sidewalk. And then the Palo Alto cops showed up. Which is when Liam failed the breathalyzer test. And they found the cocaine.

It wasn't his, but it was in the car Liam was driving. Our theory is that his friend's brother must have tucked it between the seats when he saw the police.

Rob and I got the call early Wednesday morning and had to drive down to bring him home. Rob kept quiet the whole way, which is what he always does during a crisis. And while that may work for him, it also makes it impossible for anyone else to know what he is thinking or planning on doing.

It's not a problem I suffer from.

I was worried sick as we drove into Palo Alto, and made no attempt to hide it. The police had told us over the phone that Liam had been charged with two felonies and a misdemeanor, so when we got to the station Rob started dealing with the paperwork. At the same time, one of the arresting officers drove me off to pick up Liam's car, since he wouldn't be driving it home.

When we finally got to see him, Liam was scared stiff. But with Rob on the road all the time, to say nothing of my worsening health, our eldest son didn't really have a chance. The move certainly didn't help. Maybe if I'd been strong enough to convince Rob that we were all better off in North Carolina, Liam wouldn't have fallen in with the wrong crowd. If we had passed on Big Pharma and the money and life in Silicon Valley. But I wasn't strong enough to fight my husband. I was still trying to earn love. And so, dutiful wife that I was, I just said okay and started saying goodbye to the neighbors and packing the kids' things.

I guess I fooled myself into believing that having a lot more money would make up for the disruption in the kids' lives. I really can't remember. But Rob certainly believed it. And true to his word, he started to make a lot more money. And a name for himself. While working for a company whose market value exploded. But even if he and I never talked about it, when we moved to California we both knew that Liam was headed for trouble. Our family psychologist, Dr. S., may have been a good therapist, but he saw Liam only once a week.

In the meantime, more money and more privilege and more unsupervised time translated into more opportunities for our kids to get into trouble. And one by one they all took advantage. When I was least able to help them.

And for what it's worth, when I most needed help myself.

I suppose I was learning what my mother had learned so many years ago, that becoming the sort of wife who obeyed her husband no matter what he said or did seemed like the easiest path to take at the beginning. It kept the peace. But once you gave away that big piece of yourself, you were never going to get it back. Which meant that when your kids needed you most, you'd be unable to give them a stable emotional environment. Because you'd accepted the loss of control long before. You'd accepted the passenger seat. The role of the dutiful wife. The submissive wife. The wife whose husband could do no wrong.

That's the me that my longtime friend and North Carolina neighbor Sherry saw. She didn't tell me this at the time, because she also saw that I wasn't just playing the part, I was eager to play it. And she saw that Rob loved his role too. He was the hard-working, financially successful world-renowned physician with the perfect wife.

When he was home, he'd pile the kids and their friends into the car and take them somewhere fun. Or he'd insist on me throwing a big BBQ for the neighbors where he'd play the gracious host. He never saw more than one of the kids' baseball games a year, and that only if we were lucky. But somehow, standing there on the sidelines talking to the other parents, he'd make it seem like he was a shoo-in for father-of-the-year.

In the end, it seemed my mother and I had both made the same sort of mistake. We just handled our mistakes differently. My mother reacted by working even harder than my father did, and constantly reinventing herself over the years. She threw herself into the endless work of farming, but somehow found time to earn her GED too. And she didn't stop there. She also got a diploma from a business school in Salisbury, Maryland. Then, after my father had a heart attack, she became an X-ray technician.

I gave up my career to take care of our children. And then, when my husband started traveling, I used my poor health to try to get him to pay attention to me again. And when that didn't work I took refuge in my illnesses. At the time, my family and I were living in one of the most prestigious zip codes in the country, but when the Crohn's diagnosis was added to my Addison's diagnosis, I began to have doctor appointments almost every day. And from then on, I had to care for myself first. Everyone else came second. Including our oldest, who was now facing two felonies and a misdemeanor.

Chapter Thirty

"THAT'S WAY TOO much stuff to give up all at once," I tell Xavier, unable to believe that he really expects me to stop eating red meat and bread, smoking cigarettes, and drinking diet soda.

He just looks at me without speaking, a hint of a smile on his face. Or maybe it's just a shadow that looks like a hint of a smile.

"Okay," I continue. "I can handle you telling me that I'm an abused woman. I can handle you telling me that I've been abused by the Western medical establishment, even though I'm a *part* of it. And I can accept the *possibility* that my body doesn't really need all the drugs I take. But give up my favorite foods? And diet soda too? *And* tobacco?"

He shakes his head but says nothing, his eyes never leaving mine.

"You don't understand what you're asking me to do," I plead. "Diet Coke is, well, it's like a cool breeze on a hot summer day. And freshly baked bread is a warm blanket on a cold winter night. And cigarettes are . . . well, they're like old friends stopping by for a cup of coffee and a chat."

He excuses himself. Tells me he'll be right back. I wonder if he's leaving me alone to give me time to figure it out on my own. But I've already figured it out. Giving things up isn't the real issue.

The real issue is that he's asking me to *change*.

And that scares me.

Don't get me wrong. I'm all in favor of change. I love change. Especially as an intellectual exercise. And I like it even more if the process includes some excellent massages. A little acupuncture. And some aromatic sachets.

But in order to *effect* change you have to admit that the way you've been doing things hasn't been working. In other words, that you've been wrong. For a long time. And so has everyone else. Change also means acknowledging that you have to *do* something. Something that is certain to upset the long-established equilibrium of your life. That will send vibrations across the entire universe. That will alert the powers that be that you are now willing to alter the way you live. And that's why I'm afraid.

Because you never know what change brings. Not until you do it, that is. And so as you approach the door, and reach for the handle, you find yourself wondering if you'll ever be able to walk back through it. I mean, what if you really don't like the change? Will you ever be able to return to the way things were?

Is it possible to leave the door open behind you? Or at least unlocked?

But of course it doesn't work like that. Which is why nobody wants to change. To change you need to commit. You need to pull the roller coaster's safety bar down into your lap until it clicks shut. So when the car jerks forward and begins to clatter and clank its way up the first, steep rise, there's no getting out, even though you know you're about to have the life scared out of you.

It's like leaping off the high dive. Like checking your parachute harness and then pitching yourself out of an airplane. Like leaning forward as your horse begins to take the jump.

When Xavier walks back into the treatment room I bargain with him as stubbornly as a teenager who's been told she has to clean her room before she gets her allowance. He just listens, as patient as a stone Buddha.

We slide offers back and forth across the table. I furrow my brow and cross out a couple of his demands. I add a few amendments of my own. A couple of times we reach an impasse and I push my chair back dramatically. I invoke the Bill of Rights. Basic human dignity. Xavier just sits there, impassively. Maybe even a little amused.

In the end, I agree to give up red meat, Diet Coke and bread. And I agree to buy a juicer too.

Chapter Thirty-One

I THINK EVERY MOTHER remembers her children's first steps. Maybe fathers do, too. I don't know for sure, but I do know that *my* children's first steps are locked in my memory, like clips on YouTube. First steps. First words. First little disasters.

I remember in our tiny house in the suburbs outside Washington, D.C., Liam and Nathan were down on their knees, two little boys scrubbing the hardwood floors with Comet and dish soap. "See, Mommy," says Liam, his eyes squinting with happiness. "We're helping you to clean the floor up."

I tried to smile. Didn't have the heart to tell him that after his help, we were going to have to have the floor refinished.

"Let's go for a walk," says Xavier, now that the diet negotiations have ended.

"A walk?"

"Yes," he says, "a walk. You know. One foot in front of the other. Until you're not where you used to be."

A walk. For a woman with bones as brittle as blown glass. In addition to no red meat. And a juicer. This is not going to end well. No way.

But I put my sandals on. First one, then the other.

First steps.

We head down his gravel driveway and then turn left onto the ragged asphalt road, heading west, toward the highway and the Pacific Ocean. Before we've gone fifty feet, I've had enough. "I can't do this anymore."

"Sure you can," he says, turning to look at me, but maintaining his pace.

I stop, and the space between us grows until he stops, too. "No I can't," I say. "I mean it."

My heart is pounding in my chest and my face is burning with shame, but I can't take another step. So I just stand there, defeated, and suck in ragged gasps of air while he watches.

"Let me know when you're ready," he says. A big truck goes by on the highway, and we both look.

"I'm never going to be ready," I say, taking a deep breath. "Besides, even if I were, I can't walk in these things."

Xavier looks down at my feet. I'm wearing Birkenstocks because they're the only shoes my swollen feet will fit into.

"They'll do," he says, and before I can object he puts a finger to his lips. "Ssshhh."

Once I catch my breath, we walk another short block and then cross the two-lane highway that separates his neighborhood from the coast. I stumble along after him like a little kid who can't quite match her father's stride.

Finally, on the other side of the highway, we arrive at the base of Lahilahi Point. It's really just a hill, but to my eyes it looks like a mountain. Black lava rock jutting toward the sky. Tawny grass poking out in haphazard tufts, like the poorly shaven beard of some homeless guy.

I stand there, sure that Xavier will start spouting something inspirational like, *no mountain is too high*. Or, *our only limitations are the ones we create ourselves*. I just want to go back to his house so I can get a tissue. Maybe even pick up a small piece of the self-respect I left back there on the road.

Xavier takes one last look at me and starts climbing. I stare at him in disbelief. After a few steps he turns around. "Let's go," he says, and then resumes climbing.

"Xavier, I can't."

I think to myself, is this guy crazy? I just had a walking cast removed. My seventh in fourteen months. My osteoporosis is so advanced that the simple act of walking often leads to hairline fractures. There is no way I'm going up that hill.

Xavier continues to climb.

"I really can't do this!" I call out, my voice cracking.

He turns around. "Ssshhh," he says, again, putting a finger to his lips, and then turns and continues up the hill.

I take a tentative step, my heart fluttering in my chest. I take another, and then another. My right foot slips, and I stumble and panic, wishing I could send roots down into the loose volcanic soil. "I can't do this!" I shout, Xavier's body already silhouetted against the sky. "I mean it! It's impossible!"

I choke back a sob.

Xavier's steps send a couple of small rocks tumbling down the path. I look up at him.

"Ssshhh," he says, once again, his finger to his lips, and again continues up the hill.

I can taste the salt in the air. Hear the waves lapping at the shore below us. See the gulls wheeling in the air. I clench my teeth and force myself to take a few more steps up the hill. Xavier stops every so often as I make my way up the hill. I move up via a series of stumbling lurches rather than actual steps.

"Why are you doing this to me?" I say, more to myself than him.

We finally reach a place where the hill flattens out a little. I'm sweating by now and wheezing and my thighs are killing me. Xavier points toward the edge of the plateau. I look up from my feet for the first time since we started climbing, and even though I'm here against my will, and have lived on the island for years, I'm stunned once again by the beauty of the open Pacific Ocean.

"Stand over there," he says, pointing, and for one insane moment I think he's going to tell me to jump.

And I'm so sick of all this that I probably would too. If I weren't so tired.

I move so close to the edge I can see the side of the hill fall away to the white sand beach below.

"Now look out there," he says, pointing out toward the ocean, "and tell the universe that you love yourself unconditionally."

Chapter Thirty-Two

AFTER THE FIRST Thanksgiving of the new millennium, it didn't take long to understand that the arresting officer had been right. Liam really had been very lucky. Because no one got hurt. And because it was his first offense, he got probation. Of course, he lost his driver's license. But that hurt me a lot more than it did him. Now that our first-born was finally old enough to help me ferry his brothers and sister around the valley, I was the one who ended up back behind the wheel of the family school bus.

Just as I was beginning my long journey into chronic illness.

Synthetic steroids like Prednisone are really hard to manage. They take up the slack for poorly functioning adrenal glands pretty well, but it's almost impossible to get them to mimic a healthy body's cortisol levels throughout the day. And the Crohn's made the job even harder.

My gastroenterologist, the latest addition to my growing medical team, saw it this way:

> The new diagnosis of inflammatory bowel disease certainly fits in with our suspicion of underlying auto-immune disease. It will also explain why the patient felt much better on higher doses of Prednisone. I have started her on Asacol, 400 mg. tablets at a beginning dose of two tablets t.i.d. I will see her back in about six weeks' time to check on her progress. Hopefully with

the Asacol we will be able to improve her abdominal symptoms and therefore be able to reduce her Prednisone requirement.

As an RN this all made sense to me. We were now treating the secondary disease in order to make the treatment for the primary disease more effective. The gastroenterologist's personal notes, however, were just as revealing as the report she sent my endocrinologist:

- self-adjusting her Prednisone doses
- emotionally labile
- (husband present)

Self-adjusting my synthetic steroid doses. As if I were some kid who had gotten into the medicine cabinet, not a registered nurse.

Emotionally 'labile." That's a word you hear a lot in Western medicine. Means unstable.

Husband present. Present in the medical records anyway. No wonder my ex-internist had written to him and not me in the winter of 2000, recommending that I undergo further psychiatric evaluation.

At least she was history.

Chapter Thirty-Three

I AM LITERALLY STANDING between heaven and earth, a hundred feet or so above the crashing waves, and far beneath the blue sky and its majestic clouds. Xavier settles himself on a small flat space in the volcanic rock. He's clearly been here before. And then, a slight smile on his face, he motions for me to face the water.

Is he serious? He really wants me to tell the *universe* I unconditionally love myself?

Light-headed after the climb, I try to think of a way out of this. "Couldn't I just start by telling myself?" I ask him, without turning around. "You know, in front of the mirror? At home?"

I listen for his answer but hear only the waves crashing against the rocks and the screeching of the gulls high above the shore. I add, "Maybe I could leave a note out on the counter. You know, just to remind myself."

I can almost feel his eyes on the back of my head, but I'm not going to give him the satisfaction of seeing me turn around. Instead, I gaze out over the ocean, my hair flipping around in the gusting wind.

And find myself wishing he had asked me to cluck like a chicken, crouch down and lay an egg. Because to tell you the truth, *that* would be way easier than telling the universe I love myself. Unconditionally.

I'm about to suggest the egg-laying idea when Xavier clears his throat. "Take your time," he says. "I'm not in a rush."

Angry, I turn my head in time to see him cross his legs in the lotus position. Then he lets his hands fall together in his lap and closes his eyes.

Great. Now what am I going to do? Climb back down the mountain by myself? Doesn't seem like a good idea. So I turn and stare out at the ocean. Just like he told me to. Across that infinite expanse of living water.

I still feel like crap, but it's a beautiful day. The sun is shining and banks of perfectly white clouds are sailing across the sky, reflected in the turquoise water stretching away from the white sand along the shore, until it turns to a deep blue at the horizon.

Does he realize what he's asking me to do? Does he understand that we could be here for hours? Or days, or weeks? "Look," I say, not turning around, "how would it be if I tried telling the universe that I kinda . . . sorta liked myself, maybe once a week? Say every Tuesday? And sometimes on Sundays."

No response but the crashing waves and the screeching gulls, the whistling wind and the salt in the air. "And for the record," I go on, stubbornly, "I really *did* like myself once. I think I was seven. Can't really remember why, though."

I wait for a response, and when I don't get one I sneak a look at him. He's still just sitting there on the rock, his eyes closed and his lips parting almost imperceptibly every time he exhales. Like he's not even there anymore. Like he's somewhere far from here, leaving me all alone. High above the ocean.

I turn back toward the water. Breathe the salt air in through my nose. Watch the sun sparkle on the ocean's surface, diamonds thrown out of the sea by every breaking wave. And at that moment, maybe because the view is so beautiful, it just seems unforgivably rude to disturb the universe by declaring that I unconditionally love myself. What's so important about *me*, after all?

And there's another thing too. A big thing. What if I screw up the courage to say such a crazy thing, and the universe responds: *Oh yeah? Why?*

Can't ask Xavier. He's gone somewhere far away. Just sits there with his eyes closed and his belly moving in and out, drawing air in through his nose then exhaling it through his mouth. His peacefulness irritates the hell out of me, and I turn back to look out over the ocean again. And standing there, at the edge of the cliff, more out of exhaustion than anything else, I resign myself to saying the words. Although maybe I should just think them first. Yeah. That could work.

I unconditionally love myself.

Okay, that wasn't so bad. Especially since no one could hear me say it.

My heart pounds against my ribs, the way it always does when I prepare to tell a lie. Even when I'm lying to myself.

I unconditionally love myself.

God. It sounds like the punch line of some sort of crazy cosmic joke. But I'm not laughing. Instead, tears are filling my eyes.

I *want* the words to come out. God how I want them to come out. But what is unconditional love anyway? How am I supposed to say something I don't really understand? Something I know in my heart of hearts is probably just a string of meaningless words. A stock phrase. A thing that doesn't even really exist.

Besides, my mouth is dry. My throat is like a dry well in a desert. I turn back toward Xavier, not even sure if he's still there, or if he can hear me.

"What do you say we do this tomorrow? You know, now that I know what you want me to say, there's no real hurry, is there? After all, the universe has waited this long. What's another twenty-four hours?"

"It's okay," he says, without opening his eyes. "Take your time. I don't have anything else to do today."

I sigh and again face the ocean, alone. The wind pushes tears out of my eyes.

Why is this so fucking hard? And more importantly, why is it so necessary? Can't we just double up on the acupuncture and shiatsu and throw in some herbal tea? Sing a rousing rendition of Kumbaya? Do I really have to love myself unconditionally to get well?

119

I take three, deep breaths, and then whisper the words, "I unconditionally love myself."

And whispering the words, I know right away that it's not enough. You can't whisper such powerful words. So I say them, a little louder this time. "I unconditionally love myself."

The words are a little bitter in my mouth. Metallic even. With an aftertaste of deceit.

"Again," says Xavier from his perch. "And mean it this time."

Tears slide down my cheeks. Childbirth was easier than this. Doctors and surgeries and endless medications and hospital stays were easier than this. I clench the fabric of my shirt into a wad in my fists. I close my eyes and arch my back.

"I unconditionally love myself!" I scream into the Hawaiian afternoon, the words arching through the air like arrows.

And then for reasons I don't understand, without having had the slightest expectation of any good coming from this, I feel the tiniest pinprick of light in the center of my chest. And warmth radiating from that small source.

I'm afraid to breathe again. Worried that my breath might put that tiny flame out. That firefly in the dark windy night of my illnesses.

"Okay," says Xavier. "That'll do for now."

We walk back down the hill in silence. Every so often he stops and waits for me as I make my slow way behind him. It's harder to go downhill than it was to go uphill.

Chapter Thirty-Four

ACCORDING TO NATHAN, I wasn't much of a disciplinarian when he and his brothers and sister were growing up. Which may have been true. But I was the only one of his parents who was around to give it a try. And given my childhood, I wasn't about to use my fists to establish discipline. Of course, by the fall of 2001, I had other things on my mind. Like whether I'd live to see the new year. Toward that end, a Palo Alto pulmonologist was added to my team.

Excerpts from his first report, which was forwarded to my endocrinologist, are below.

> ... patient with Addison's disease, micro-Crohn's disease, and previous ovarian vein thrombosis. I deliberately lift these out, because I think that if I were smart enough, this would tell me her pulmonary diagnosis.

In other words, my pulmonologist wasn't, as he put it, "smart enough" to come up with a solid pulmonary diagnosis from my history alone, although I gave him credit for admitting that. He went on to write:

> Also, when I saw her on 9/17/01 I explicitly discussed with her the importance of stopping smoking. As you know, she

smokes approximately ten cigarettes per day. I gave her some of the basic informational material on tobacco dependency, diagnosis, and treatment. She has set a target quit date for 10/7/01.

I wish I had more to offer, but hopefully we will be able to get to the bottom of this.

Chapter Thirty-Five

"Y OU KNOW," SAYS Xavier, as I lie on his treatment table, a couple of weeks after our climb up the hill, "some indigenous peoples believe that disease has as much to do with an imbalance in the tribal dynamic as it does with a person's own health. They think that to restore balance and eliminate disease, it's sometimes necessary for a person who is ill to leave the tribe."

Is this guy on drugs? How'd we get from telling the universe I unconditionally love myself to leaving the tribe?

"Then, once he or she is outside the environment in which they became ill, it's easier to see what's going wrong, and to adopt a different, healthier lifestyle."

What? Is he asking me to move away from my family now?

Xavier continues to slide acupuncture needles into my body. "Your family dynamic is a big part of what's made you sick," he says, "and what *keeps* you sick. So, if you really want to heal . . ."

". . . of course, I want to heal . . ."

". . . well then, you're going to have to remove yourself from the environment that's fostered your illnesses. It's as simple as that."

Xavier continues to discuss diet with me. And the effect diet has on the body, which he maintains is essentially a self-correcting mechanism. But, he says, for the body to self-correct or to heal, certain conditions must be met. "No one can heal in a toxic environment," he tells me at the end of another session.

"You mean, like living next to a nuclear power plant, or something like that?"

He shakes his head. "No, I don't mean that at all, and you know it. We've talked about this before. I'm talking about your family, and how continuing to live with them is keeping you from healing."

I let that one sink in for a bit.

"Okay, but what am I supposed to do? Kick them out of the house?"

"Or find your own space."

"By myself? That's how I'm going to heal?"

He nods serenely.

"But I hate being alone."

"You'll get used to it," Xavier says. "In fact, you might even learn to appreciate it one day."

"Don't hold your breath," I tell him.

Which was a little stupid, I have to admit, because if there's one thing this man knows how to do, it's control his breathing.

Okay. I won't deny my family has boundary issues. In fact, the central issue is that there are no boundaries. And I'm probably the worst offender.

We're twisted together like skeins of yarn after a litter of kittens gets ahold of them. You can't tell where one family member ends and another begins. Just one big tangle. Psychologists call this *enmeshment*. And just like Xavier, they consider it an unhealthy way to live. Even if you do it to satisfy the needs of others, the point remains that it's not good for *you*.

"I'd love to live on my own for a while," I finally tell Xavier. "Keep everyone in my family out of the house until I begin to feel better. Especially because it's really going to piss them off."

So, I do what I said I would. I leave the tribal environment. Again. Because I've already left the house in Northern California, the tribal environment I got sick in. But since I'm already in Hawaii, I don't go far. Just across the driveway that separates our two houses in Kaneohe Bay. I move out of the white house, where we spent our first family vacations on the island, to the yellow house, which we bought as a rental property next door. Liam and his girlfriend Allison have just moved out. They're on their way to Chicago, where Liam will begin law school.

Moving into the new house is not easy. I'm still not sure I wouldn't rather be sick in the tribe than be well outside of it. The tribe is all I've ever had. All I've ever known. All I've ever wanted.

A little paranoid, I imagine that whenever Rob's in Hawaii, he and Cat and Cole huddle around the kitchen table in the white house and grumble about Xavier. They've been doing a lot of that lately. They're probably daring each other right now to cross the driveway and ring the doorbell under some pretense. Just to see if I'm serious about not letting them in.

I *am* serious. Even though I hate hiding out in the yellow house. Way too big for one person. I feel like I'm some crazy old actress in a movie. Like Xavier is asking me to choose between my health and my family. Well, I want both.

Not that he cares. "You're not as important to them as you think you are. Just focus on yourself and your family will find a new equilibrium."

Easy for him to say. He doesn't have any kids.

I almost feel like I'm holding myself hostage. And if that's the case, is anyone going to be willing to pay the ransom?

Chapter Thirty-Six

B Y THE SPRING of 2002, in northern California, five different subspecialists were being copied on my medical reports. And a growing number of those reports were coming from my pulmonologist.

> CURRENT MEDICATIONS: Prednisone 20 mg, qd.; Pulmicort, 800 mcg (4 doses), q12h; Prevacid 30-60 mg, qd.; Florinef, 0.1 mg, qd.; Fosamax, 70 mg, 1 tablet qweek: Calcium, 600 mg, qd.; Soy capsules, 2 capsules qd.; DHEA, 10 mg, 1 gel cap qd.; Salt tablets, 1 PRN

> PHYSICAL EXAMINATION: WEIGHT: 162 pounds (up 5.5 pounds from 13 days ago. BMI:24.6 (upper end of the healthy weight range). BLOOD PRESSURE: 118/70. HEART RATE: 96 and regular. RESPIRATIONS: 12 and unlabored. TEMPERATURE: 98.4 F.

A few months later, in July of 2002, yet another gastroenterologist, who was an expert in inflammatory bowel disease, described my condition this way.

> In summary, this is a complicated 40-year-old woman with a constellation of disease. She has Crohn's disease of the colon,

bronchiectasis, and Addison disease. The question is whether all three of these diseases are related. Ulcerative colitis has been associated in one case report with Addison disease.

I'd gone way past being a member of the Patient-of-the-Month Club. This was Patient-of-the-Day stuff. Sometimes even Patient-of-the-Hour stuff. So naturally it was time for us to move again.

Not that I was unwilling. Rob and I had had our eyes on a place for some time, a much bigger Spanish-style house on almost three acres. Built for an artist, with interior arches and handmade Mexican tile, it had been on the market for a while. The house needed some work. By no means ostentatious by the standards of our suburb, it was still a big improvement over our tiny place on the other side of the hill. It had a tennis court, a neglected swimming pool, plenty of room for a garden and a greenhouse for flowers too. But most importantly, room enough for two growing teenage boys and two middle schoolers. And me and Rob. So despite my declining health, we bought it and started renovations.

In those days, it seemed that whenever Rob was in town he wanted to throw a big party for his colleagues and their wives. Business was good in Big Pharma and everybody wanted to show off. You needed a house featured in Architectural Digest. A slim, tanned, trophy wife. A cellar packed with the world's finest wines.

Well, I guess two out of three would have to do. Which was too bad since I didn't drink. But Rob and his friends sure did. And so did our older boys.

The move was definitely a good thing. But my handling it alone while I was sick, and Rob was on the road, was a little like asking Atlas to hold up two globes at once. Still, somehow I managed. And then finished the year up by fracturing three ribs in a fall.

Chapter Thirty-Seven

X AVIER WON'T STOP talking about diet. "You need a steady stream of natural, unprocessed, easily digestible nutrients," he says. "That way your body will free up the energy it wastes digesting heavy foods and use that energy to heal itself."

Well, I'd bought a juicer. Just like I said I would. I just hadn't gotten around to using it. In fact, just taking it out of the box was hard enough for me. Plus there was no one around to help me put it together. Finally, it struck me as more than a little strange that this enormous, electrified metal contraption was the secret to a healthy "natural" diet. Did all those indigenous people he loves to talk about just run out and buy one at a department store in the jungle?

Either way the juicer still sits there on the kitchen counter. Like it's sulking. Which I'm doing a little of myself. Out on the lanai with a lit cigarette in one hand.

I'll quit tomorrow.

It's December and I'm still off bread and Diet Coke. Mostly. Eliminating meat isn't really a problem. It's been causing me digestive trouble for years. But no point in telling Xavier that. Better he should think I'm giving something up.

In the meantime I add more greens to my diet. And more fresh fruits. I also experiment with nuts and seeds like Xavier suggested.

I eat oatmeal with blueberries and flax seed oil for breakfast, a combination that some people think inhibits the growth of cancer. Sautéed beet greens with roasted tomatoes and pine nuts for lunch. Vegetable ratatouille for dinner. And I see Xavier for treatments three times a week.

A few weeks after I lock my family out of my house, I start letting them back in. At least the ones who are on the island. Nathan is already studying at the University of Colorado. Liam is in Chicago. Rob is rarely here. So I let Cat and Cole in, but only on my terms. I need all my energy for healing, I tell them. So no drama, please. And no demands.

And no snack food, alcohol or tobacco either. To make the point I put an "amnesty" box outside the front door. You know, like the ones the TSA have before you go through security. A place you can leave the stuff you're not supposed to carry onto a plane before boarding.

The truce is an uneasy one, but we manage to remain civil. At first. They ask how I'm doing. Stare at me like I'm a vaguely familiar animal. One they've seen in a zoo, or on TV, that may or may not have become dangerous. This is okay, I guess. I find myself looking at them in pretty much the same way.

So much for Mother of the Year. But like Xavier says, it's a process.

Unfortunately, the process seems to include deep dark depressions. They wind their way into the yellow house like fog seeping in through an open window. And if I don't watch out, they wrap me in wet gray wool and drag me down into the depths.

Taking myself off Humira probably has something to do with it. Which means I'm down to only eleven medications. Only eleven medications. For the first time in ten years I begin to see just how absurd that number of meds is. Especially since I don't experience any major Crohn's flare-ups when I go off Humira. Just the usual cycle of depression.

"Don't fight it, just *sit* with the depression," Xavier tells me gently. "Observe it, and try to let it flow through you."

"Let it flow through me?" I ask him in response. "It feels like I'm wading through an ocean of it."

He smiles. "Depression, like every illness, has something to teach you."

"Well, I've learned enough for one day, thank you very much. In fact, I've learned enough for a whole month."

He shakes his head.

"Stop complaining and try to be grateful."

This is not the first time I've heard that statement.

"You always make such a big deal out of everything," Xavier tells me. And then I tell him he's wrong. And then a few minutes later I find myself crying and shouting and stomping my feet. Or, to put it another way, making his point for him.

We're sitting at the picnic table in his backyard after a treatment. It's late afternoon and he is feeding me seaweed salad with a pair of chopsticks. "Seaweed," he says, "is good for the thyroid. It's loaded with iodine, and the thyroid needs iodine to function properly."

I'd rather take a pill, but I keep that to myself.

It's not a good day. The tears just won't stop. I'm in the grip of a sadness so deep that my bones ache. I can barely breathe. I haven't eaten well for a couple of days, by which I mean I really haven't been eating at all.

"That's no way to build trust with your body," says Xavier. "You have to nurture it, not neglect it."

And as he talks, he continues to feed me seaweed, like a mother spoon-feeding an infant. With chopsticks.

"What happened to set you off this time?" he asks, without the slightest sign of sympathy. As if he's asking me about the weather.

"Nothing in particular. Things are all right, really. Smooth even. I'm getting along with the kids. When I see them. And getting along with Rob, too. Not that I see much of him, either. But what did I expect, working with a healer who tells me I have to isolate myself like some kind of a monk."

"You wouldn't last a week as a monk," says Xavier.

"Good," I respond. "I'd rather draw. Stay up with my art classes. Write in my journal." My voice cracks.

"Until the next hole opens up inside me, and every good feeling is sucked into it."

Xavier dips the chopsticks back into the bowl of seaweed, then raises a dripping blob of the translucent greens to my lips. I keep my mouth shut tight. Shake my head like a stubborn toddler.

"Come on," he says, making gentle, green circles in front of my mouth. "Don't be such a drama queen."

"I am *not* a drama queen," I respond, then take the seaweed into my mouth.

God, I hate this stuff. It's not just the taste. It's the texture too. I think its closest botanical relative has got to be rubber. It squeaks while I chew.

"You *are* a drama queen," Xavier says. "You have a pathological need for attention, and drama brings attention."

I nearly choke on my seaweed.

"Face it," he says, unconcerned by my blocked airway. "You're an addict, and one of the things you're addicted to is drama. And the depression and the anxiety you're feeling now are classic signs of withdrawal."

Like any good addict, after thinking it over, I open with an outraged denial. "I am not addicted to drama," I tell Xavier, as he pinches another glob of seaweed between the chopsticks. "And I don't go around seeking attention."

"Then how do you explain that pack of doctors?" he asks. "How many subspecialists do you have? How many therapists?"

I try to add them up but keep losing count. "Not that many."

He huffs through his nose.

"Okay," I say, "there are six of them. Plus the other two, but they're not involved all the time."

"Eight doctors," he says. "And you're not addicted to attention?"

"I need those doctors, and you know it. What I don't need is more seaweed," I say, and struggle to my feet.

Xavier walks me to the truck. "Accept that you're an addict, and stop fighting the depression," he says. "Just let it do its work, but don't get all twisted up in it. Try to think of it as a fever for the soul. You need the heat right now, but as long as you don't cling to it, it will pass."

He gives me a hug. "Now go home and make yourself some juice."

I say thanks and ease myself into the car.

When I get home I walk right past the juicer, crawl into bed, pull the covers over my head and start to cry.

Chapter Thirty-Eight

BY LATE 2003, several of my physicians were encouraging me to think about fundoplication surgery, because of my worsening gastroesophageal reflux disease, also known as GERD. The procedure is done laparoscopically. Which means it's non-invasive. The doctors just make a small incision and insert the necessary instruments instead of opening you all the way up. Either way, the goal of fundoplication is wrapping the uppermost portion of the stomach around the esophagus to prevent gastric reflux.

Below is an excerpt from my pulmonologist's report dated December 15, 2003.

I told her that this is the first time, ever, in my professional career as a pulmonologist that I have actually recommended fundoplication or surgical intervention for GERD. In her case, I think that is warranted. I think that such surgery, if it is successful, will not only alleviate the dysphagia that she has but also eliminate the episodic, diffuse anterior chest pain that she experiences, which I believe is secondary to airway bronchoconstriction and inflammation when GERD flares.

She is also using her treadmill six to seven days per week. She uses it between 4-7 miles per house, at 0% grade, for a minimum of 1 mile (that takes her 30-40 minutes) to 5-6 miles per hour (that would take her between 60-90 minutes).

Tobacco dependence: 100% tobacco-free since 10/25/02

The report ends with these words.

> Overall . . . I continue to be really pleased with the progress Mrs. R. is making. She is too.

He was right. I was pleased with my progress too. For a while anyway. And I went ahead with the arthroscopic fundoplication surgery in March of 2004. But the multiple medications, and especially the Enbrel, were beginning to wreak havoc on my body. In June of 2004 I saw my pulmonologist again, and he noted the following in the report he sent to my endocrinologist.

> Because of concern of lymphoma as a possible side effect from Enbrel, in mid-April she decided to discontinue Enbrel. Unfortunately she has noted, since doing so, that she has had slow progressive worsening of Crohn's disease, various joint pains and aches, as well as chest tightness.
>
> She is also very concerned about the highly abnormal fasting lipid panel which you obtained on 4/29/04. As you know, she has, apparently, a very bad family history of coronary artery disease. She continues to use her treadmill 6-7 days per week, going a 3-4 mph at a 0% grade for a minimum of 1 mile up to a maximum of 3-4 miles.

I never really liked walking the treadmill, because no matter how many steps you take you never go anywhere. But I liked the idea of a heart attack even less.

Chapter Thirty-Nine

XAVIER TALKS A lot about our natural resistance to change. After a particularly stubborn episode of mine, complete with tears, he again walks me down Makaha Valley Road toward the ocean. Once more we cross the highway, but this time we walk out onto the beach. Nothing but white sand and the blue-green ocean in front of us. Pastel blue sky above it all, and waves curling in toward the shore.

Xavier draws a line in the sand and motions for me to stand on one side of it. Then he stands on the other side so we're facing each other. Finally, he takes my left elbow in his right hand. I do the same to him, and then we clasp our free hands between us.

"Now," he says. "Push as hard as you can."

Of course he's stronger than I am. But I weigh almost two hundred pounds. And I'm mad at the world. So even with all the pushing and groaning, we each stay on our side of the line.

"You're not trying," he says, releasing his grip. He takes a new stance and reaches for my elbow again. And this time, fueled by anger, I push with everything I've got, and he simply steps to one side and allows me to tumble forward into the sand.

I'm not happy when I get up.

"The point," he says, smiling with his eyes, "is not to meet resistance. Just let it go past you."

I brush my arms off. I didn't make the long drive to Makaha to play in the sand. Or to take an Aikido lesson either.

"You can't fight resistance head-on," he continues, slowly repeating the sidestep he'd taken a moment earlier. "But with a very small shift, you can allow the powerful energy of resistance to slip harmlessly past you."

I'm sure he's right, but I'm just not in the mood for this. My gaze drifts, finding Lahilahi Point. Rising directly behind Xavier. He seems to know what I'm thinking, but after a look over one shoulder, he begins to walk back toward the highway. No climbing today.

"You don't always have to climb a mountain to talk to the universe," he says as we make our way back to his place.

"Then why'd you make me do it?" I ask, breathing heavily.

"Because you use your diseases as an excuse. As an excuse not to challenge yourself."

I let that one sink in. "So, now you're saying that I could have just stood there in my own backyard and told the universe that I love myself unconditionally?"

"Of course you could have. But by getting up that little hill you proved to yourself that you could do something you thought you couldn't."

Great. But he seems to have forgotten that I never *wanted* to climb that hill. What I'd like to do, instead, is lose the steroid hump on my back. And if all this mumbo-jumbo won't help me do that, then what am I doing here?

But I don't ask that question, because I already know the answer. I guess I'm starting to realize that Xavier's right, even if I can't quite admit it yet. In order to heal I have to learn to care for *myself*. Which, just like climbing that hill, is something I never really tried to do. Ever. Because I never thought I could.

Chapter Forty

PATIENTS JOKE ALL the time about doctors' handwriting, how it looks more like hieroglyphics than English. But as my medical records piled up over the years it wasn't the handwritten notes that surprised me, it was the number of simple mistakes. Like misspelled medications or diseases. Errors in grammar. Or worst of all, confusion about just who was being treated.

Every one of these errors surfaced in an assessment written in November of 2004 by an Associate Professor of Clinical Medicine at a teaching hospital in San Francisco. By then, my medical team had been treating my chronic illnesses for more than four and half years. And I was beginning to feel more and more divorced from my own treatment. I felt as if I had become an old woman sitting in the corner while everybody else in the family sat down to a big noisy dinner. Present, but neither seen nor heard nor spoken to.

I think it makes excellent sense to switch her from Enbrel to another anti-TNF agent that has the potential to both treat her inflammatory bowel disease as well as her joint problems. The two choices would be Remicade or Humira. Humira benefits from its ease of use in that it is a subcutaneous injection, much like Enbrel . . . although I would still rate Remicade as the first line agent for Crohn.

It's Crohn's disease. Not Crohn. And as an RN I couldn't help but wonder what it meant that my own doctor didn't even care enough to call my diseases by their correct names. But the following paragraph was the one that really got to me.

> I had a long talk about the risks and benefits of these medications, and certainly, the risk profile is not terribly different than that of Enbrel. The patient and his wife . . .

Yeah. That's right. Referring to Rob and me the doctor wrote "the patient and his wife." More than four years into the treatment of my chronic illnesses I had somehow been moved to the periphery. In this doctor's eyes Rob was now the patient. If you believe in Freudian slips that is.

> The patient and his wife are quite concerned about the long half-life of Remicade because of the risk of infection given her Addison disease and are more inclined to use a medication that might be easier to terminate if needed.

He was right about that at least. We were worried about what might happen if the Remicade caused more problems than it solved. Because it stays in the blood for weeks.

In early December of 2005, my pulmonologist set up a lunch meeting with seven of my doctors. A meeting "devoted to sorting out the next steps of what to do for Mrs. R. . . . so we can optimally treat this woman who has more medical conditions than any person twice her age has the right to have."

My doctors had my best interests at heart, I'm sure of that. And what they were doing made sense to me as a nurse. Plus Rob was involved. But we were more than five years into their aggressive campaign to manage my multiple illnesses and we hadn't even succeeded in my managing my *symptoms*.

So I started to lose faith. Or maybe it was just that the medications and their side effects had finally caught up with me.

140

Part IV
Healing

Chapter Forty-One

"HAVE YOU EVER considered the possibility that your medications are clouding your judgment?" Xavier asks me.

The question comes out of nowhere, as we're walking down the beach. "Well, it doesn't really matter whether my meds are clouding my judgment or not," I say, irritated by the question. "If I don't take them I'll die . . ."

". . . and you'll also die if you do. We're *all* going to die. What I'm asking you is a completely different question. I'm asking you how you want to *live*, and whether you can answer that question while you're on drugs."

As if I had a choice. "How would I like to live? I'd like to live without joint pain, fevers, clogged up sinuses and a heartbeat like a hamster's."

"And what exactly is keeping you from doing that?"

For a moment, I feel like I'm talking to Rob. Or to my father. Like there are things I just can't understand, and so, as a good little girl I just do as I'm told. "My illnesses are keeping me from living like that, obviously."

"Your illnesses," Xavier responds, "or your treatment?"

Ah, the men in my life. I'm almost fifty years old, and just beginning to recognize the pattern.

My father didn't treat me and my mother and sister and brother as if we were his family. He treated us more like we were his responsibilities. Responsibilities like the ones he had at work, without any emotional connection. Controlling us not for control's sake, but because it was easier for him to live up to his responsibilities that way.

My physician husband treats me like I'm the sole subject of some sort of personal research project of his. It's like our relationship is something he does on the side when he's not out in the world saving lives. And sleeping with other women. The boys treat me like a maid.

Xavier treats me like a child.

The wind picks up. Gulls shriek high above us. Small waves slap the shore as gently and rhythmically as hands on a drum.

Okay. That's not really fair. Xavier treats me like a child with great powers. Which isn't really the same thing at all. But he also says I haven't learned how to use those powers. Or more accurately, how to get out of their way and just let them work. As if it's all so easy.

"So, what you're saying is, all I have to do is quit taking my medications and I'll be fine?"

"I didn't say that," he responds. "Listen to your body, and it will let you know when you no longer need the drugs. I'm just asking you if it isn't possible that, after all these years, your medications might be preventing you from seeing who you really are, what you're really doing to yourself, and where the road you're on is taking you."

We walk another five or ten minutes in silence, and then he stops and faces the ocean. "You know the difference between swimming on the mainland and swimming on the island?"

Oh Jesus, here we go again. Another question right out of the blue, because neither one of us have been talking about swimming. In fact we've *never* talked about swimming. But once he gets going, there's no stopping him. "On the mainland," he continues, "you swim laps in a pool, right? You just go back and forth and back and forth and back and forth."

"Okay," I say, not really interested in helping him make his point.

"In the open ocean, it's different. Let's say, for instance, that you

146

swim from Lahilahi down to Kaneilio," he says, pointing south, in the direction of Waianae.

"Okay, let's say you do."

"You start by swimming *away* from where you are," he says, looking me in the eyes. "And that's only natural. But there's a point, somewhere out there," he says, pointing toward the open water, "where you stop swimming *away* from something and begin to swim *toward* something."

We walk another quarter mile or so along the shore before I can finally admit he's right. To myself, that is. I've been swimming *away* from something for most of my life.

Chapter Forty-Two

B Y 2006, MY doctors were meeting for lunch every month. They still hadn't been able to stabilize my rapidly-shifting physical ailments, to say nothing of my emotional state, but they were better able to coordinate their treatments and the resulting side effects. This was even more important after 2005 when a third life-threatening autoimmune disease showed up in my bloodwork.

Diabetes mellitus, Type 2.

When you've been on corticosteroids as long as I had your immune system becomes suppressed. It's what the steroids are designed to do. Or you could look at it this way. To keep your body from attacking itself, you need to shut down the system designed to protect your body from outside attack.

At the time of my Type 2 diabetes diagnosis, I was on three different kinds of synthetic corticosteroids: Prednisone, which lasts anywhere from six to eight hours; Cortef, which is short-acting and which I used only when I suffered from tachycardia or when my blood pressure dropped; and Dexamethasone, which is the longest acting of the three and which can reduce the highs and lows of both blood sugar and blood pressure. Dexamethasone is most often given to people who have sustained heavy brain trauma. I took one milligram every day, which may have set the stage for my diabetes. And the fluctuations in my blood sugar further derailed my immune system.

Around that time, an old friend from our early days in California came down from Seattle for a visit. Her most vivid memory at that time was of me sitting in the living room with a calculator trying to figure out how big a dose of steroids to give myself. After taking into consideration what I'd had to eat, of course, and when, and how much insulin I'd already taken.

Of course my doctors had to react to my latest diagnosis too.

> She [Julie] has been on oral glucose controlling medications but unfortunately has not had any success. She was advised to start insulin in the last two weeks . . . blood work shows a white count of 1.27, platelet count 465, and a glucose of 162. The [low] white count is likely due to her chronic steroid use which is now 35 mg of Prednisone a day.

By the summer of 2006, eight and sometimes nine doctors were being copied on the most routine reports. And every time a new doctor was asked to consult, a new history had to be assembled. For example, a new gastroenterologist saw me this way.

> On physical examination this is a very pleasant, but depressed-appearing middle-age woman who is obviously cushingoid, who is alert and oriented in no apparent distress.
>
> In summary, Ms. R. is a 45-year-old, very complicated woman . . . I spent a long time discussing with Ms. R. and her husband regarding her condition and I told her very frankly that as far as I can tell she had a very thorough and thoughtful workup by a team of highly qualified physicians to date.

I gave them every opportunity to continue to showcase their diagnostic skills. In 2006 I had three separate sinus surgeries. The year 2007 began with a cholecystectomy, which is the surgical removal of the gallbladder. A few months after that surgery, I developed acute pyelonephritis, an inflammation of the kidneys, most likely brought on by a urinary tract infection. That led to a new regimen of antibiotics and a two-week stay in the hospital.

But those were just footnotes to my autoimmune diseases, which by 2008 included yet another. Hypothyroidism.

The risk for hypothyroidism increases greatly if you suffer from other autoimmune diseases. It begins with lowered thyroid production. Something like Addison's begins with lower cortisol production, and if left untreated, it usually proceeds to the destruction of the thyroid gland itself.

Liam couldn't help commenting on my reaction to the news, which was so different from everyone else's. "Do you realize, Mom, how happy you are whenever you find out you have a new disease?"

Chapter Forty-Three

I REACH THE LAST page of the 2010 calendar. December's grid, not dotted with nearly as many medical notes and appointments as it used to be. Above it is a photograph of a rural landscape blanketed with snow.

None of that here on Oahu.

Three months have passed since I started working with Xavier. Am I getting better? I don't know. I do feel a little different. But at this time of the year it might be nothing more than the Christmas spirit, which strangely enough works its magic in Hawaii just as surely as it does on the mainland. And like everyone else young or old, I occasionally wonder what I'll find under the tree.

As it turns out my first gift is a dog bite.

The holidays approach. We're all sitting at the dining room table in Oahu when it happens. Cat, Cole, and Nathan too, in from Colorado. Liam has also flown in from Chicago with Allison.

Quality family time. Until little Beatrice comes racing under the table, with Liam's much bigger dog Buddha right behind her. Without thinking, I throw my leg up to block Buddha, and leading with his teeth he accidentally shears a piece of skin off my leg.

An accident pure and simple. If you believe in accidents.

I think I've said it somewhere before, but two of the more damaging side-effects of long-term steroid use are decreased resistance to infection, and skin that becomes paper thin. In fact after ten years of synthetic steroids, my skin was about as tough as the wrapping paper on the gifts stacked under the tree. And almost as brightly decorated, too, if you count all the bruises, scars, cuts and bandages.

But there are ways for me to deal with an infection. The most important thing is to keep my corticosteroid levels from bottoming out. If they get too low, my entire metabolic machine grinds to a halt. And I die. So I always carry injectable steroids with me. Just in case.

But that isn't the most dangerous aspect of the bite. Instead, the problem is the effect of my diabetes, because fluctuations in my blood sugars further derail the immune system. So any kind of open wound takes much longer to heal, if it heals at all. And if it doesn't heal, it's possible that my leg might have to be amputated below the knee. Unlikely, but possible. Just think about the people you've seen with Diabetes type 2 who've suffered the loss of an arm or a leg.

As these cheerful holiday thoughts occupy my mind, the dogs, yelping and snapping, their claws skittering across the tile floor, finally disappear down the hall. I look down at my wound and see blood pooling on the floor beneath me.

All hell breaks loose around me. Cat's screams are louder than the others. "We have to get you to the hospital!"

I gaze down at the open, bleeding wound on my leg. Looks like somebody flayed part of my shin with a sharp knife. And looking at it, my trauma nurse training kicks in, and I start giving my children instructions. For some reason I insist that the blood has to be cleaned up before we leave. Which is really idiotic given how precarious my situation is. I *do* need to get to the hospital. Time is of the essence. But there is something intoxicating about the chaos.

And no one knows where Rob is.

Given the condition of my skin, the best the doctors can do is sew the pieces of torn flesh together with giant Raggedy-Ann sutures. They're the only kind my skin will hold. Then they wrap my leg in gauze and bandages and send us home with peroxide and antibiotics and strict instructions on how to keep the wound clean. I don't even bother telling them I'm a nurse.

When we get back to the white house, I call Xavier and tell him

154

what happened. He laughs. "What's so funny," I ask him, "about a trip to the emergency room?"

"You'll be fine," he says, still trying to keep himself from laughing.

"I don't see anything funny about it."

"You want to know what's funny? You still saying you're not addicted to drama."

Xavier drives across the island anyway to survey the damage, and then watches as I carefully unwrap the bandage and remove the gauze.

"Sometimes you need the dog to bite you," he says, nodding thoughtfully.

He leaves and Rob shows up. I tell him what my Eastern healer said and he throws a red-faced tantrum.

Part of me is delighted. He still cares. There's still hope for our marriage.

"I don't care what this Xavier character says," Rob tells me. "You can forget about curing Addison's disease with diet, incense and massage."

As ridiculous as it sounds, his anger sends a thrill through me. Is it possible he still loves me? Is it possible he still cares? Even though it looks like he's married to the hunchback of Notre Dame?

Because I still want him to care. I still want that badly, more than anything else. Even if I have to be bitten by dogs for us to find our way back to each other. Even if Xavier's right and I *am* addicted to drama. It doesn't matter. Because at this moment I feel closer to my husband than I have in a long, long time.

A few days later Rob flies off to some pharmaceutical conference somewhere. Nathan gets on a flight to the mainland. Liam and Allison fly back to Chicago. The others, who have to start classes again at Hawaii Pacific, return to their routines.

Alone again.

I know. Whining.

I'm spending far too many hours on the couch in the clutches of self-pity and loneliness. Withdrawal symptoms? I don't know. But

Xavier's right about one thing. I'd much rather have some drama around here.

Still, I manage to take care of myself, to routinely clean my wound. Every morning, every noon and every night I unwind the bandage. Hoist my leg up on a chair. Take off the layer of gauze netting, remove that awful pad and douse the wound with foaming peroxide. Slather the wound again with greasy antibiotics and place a fresh white piece of gauze over it. Wrap that with still more gauze. Then twine the bandage around my calf again.

And something starts to happen in those quiet moments of self-care.

I begin to learn how to be gentle with *myself*. To nurture *myself*. And at that moment I begin to believe that caring for *myself* just might be possible. It's a long-awaited, brief moment of clarity. Maybe the house isn't so empty after all.

I'm still here.

Chapter Forty-Four

IN 2007, SEVEN years into my odyssey among the autoimmune diseases, I was on the verge of collapse. But I still took short trips to Oahu whenever I could. Mostly I went to get out of California more than anything else, although I wanted to check in on Liam and Cole too. Which meant that I ended up at the Medical Center in Kailua more and more often. And that meant that the staff at Kailua got to write their own chapter of my ongoing medical history.

PAST MEDICAL HISTORY: Significant for Crohn [sic] disease, primary Addison's disease, type 2 diabetes mellitus, asthma, melanoma 1979, history of 2 gastrointestinal bleeds 1980, and bronchiectasis with ground glass opacities of the lungs 2001. The patient has a history of kidney stones x2 in 1978 with calcium oxalate stone.

FAMILY HISTORY: Noncontributory.

SOCIAL HISTORY: The patient denies any alcohol or recreational drug use. She is married to an infectious disease physician and lives in California.

CURRENT MEDICATIONS:

1. Prednisone 20 mg 1 tablet daily
2. Florinef 0.05, 1 tablet daily

3. Avandia 5 mg 1 tablet daily
4. DHEA 25 mg 1 tablet daily
5. Wellbutrin XL 300 mg 1 tablet daily
6. Allegra 60 mg 1 tablet twice daily
7. Calcium 600 mg 1 tablet twice daily
8. Metformin 1000 mg 1 tablet daily
9. Lipitor 20 mg 1 tablet p.o. daily

GENERAL: The patient is a pleasant Caucasian female with cushingoid appearance in no acute distress.

By then my long list of medications no longer seemed unusual to me. I was sick, so naturally I needed a lot of meds. And I just had to forget as well as I could the inevitability of side effects and drug-related complications. My doctors weren't concerned, nor was my husband, and given that I was a nurse first, and a patient second, I saw no reason to worry either.

Back in California, I consulted with yet another associate professor from the university hospital.

As you know, the patient is a delightful 46-year-old nurse with apparent Crohn's disease and history of recent abnormal liver biochemistries. She came to clinic today with her husband, who is quite supportive. The history below was obtained from the patient and her husband (they are very good historians) as well as my review of approximately 50 pages of office notes, laboratory, radiological, and histological data.

His report ran to nine pages. There were nineteen separate conditions or incidents listed under my recent medical history. He concluded his report honestly enough by writing that he had "relatively few recommendations regarding this patient's care at the current time." But in the event of "persistently elevated liver biochemistries," he advised us to consider a liver biopsy.

In late June of 2007 I made a follow-up visit to my pulmonologist.

Her pulmonary function tests were highly abnormal and substantially worse than the previous studies of 12/8/06.

She also indicated she is planning to start Humira, as soon as her husband will be around. I thought it was reasonable for her to delay that until he is around. He has been doing a tremendous amount of traveling the last couple weeks but does plan to be home over the next few weeks.

Twelve other doctors were copied.

Chapter Forty-Five

SOMETHING ELSE HAPPENS to me during the weeks after the dog bite. Maybe because I can't do much besides limp between the kitchen, the lanai, and the living room. So, it seems like a good time to just think. And what I think about is the way Xavier continues to describe me. Matter of factly, and without the slightest emotion.

"You're an addict, Julie. And you're not only addicted to drama, you're addicted to drugs, too." It takes me a long time to confront those blunt accusations. Like walking past a mirror over and over again before finally stopping to take a look at yourself, knowing you're not going to like what you see. But as the waters muddied by my self-delusion finally begin to clear I catch a glimpse of myself as I am. See myself as he does. For a second or two anyway. Before turning away in embarrassment.

"Why is that so hard for you to admit?" Xavier asks me when we talk next, sounding really surprised. "You're a registered nurse, your husband works in the drug industry, and you're unwell. What else did you think was going to happen?"

He's right of course. But it's one thing for him to be right and another thing for me to admit it. Especially since my mind is so accustomed to falling back on the same old justifications.

"Okay, but it's not like we're not talking about crystal meth or heroin here," I say. "These are *medications* I'm taking, not *drugs*. They were prescribed by licensed . . ."

161

"... by licensed drug dealers," he says, finishing the sentence for me. "And you've been one of their best customers for years."

Years and years is more like it, although there's no point in telling *him* that. Okay, it wasn't coke or heroin, but it was still some heavy-duty stuff. And I had been taking it day after day, month after month, and year after year.

"Okay. I admit that I'm *dependent* on my medications. But that's not the same thing as being a drug addict."

"What's the difference?" he asks me, in that infuriatingly straight-forward way of his. Like he's really trying to understand.

"The difference," I say, sounding like a snotty teenager, "is that if I get pulled over the police can't arrest me."

He shakes his head. "You're doing it again. Creating the most dramatic scenario possible ..."

"... no I'm not. I'm just making the point that my medications are legal."

"Call it what you will, but you're still swimming *away* from something. Instead of *toward* something."

He's really starting to get annoying. What happened to acupuncture and massage? To soothing floral sachets?

Okay. I admit it. I'm a drug addict. And I'm addicted to drama too.

But I'm not going to admit it out loud. Not yet, anyway. And definitely not to *him*.

The drama makes me feel alive. And what's wrong with that? Besides it's not just me. We all need drama. It gives our lives texture and dimensionality. And personally I need it like I need air. Without it, I think I'd simply disappear.

I've known this since I was a little girl. It was how my family operated. There was never a place set for calmness at our table. And if by some chance there was a moment or two of peace, you could be sure that storm clouds were gathering on the horizon. Dark and foreboding. Like an undertaker parked in front of a home where someone was ill. Waiting for the inevitable.

Chapter Forty-Six

As 2011 BEGINS, my focus continues to turn inward. Probably because I'm spending more time on my own than I ever have before. Not that I like it, because I don't. It's the one thing I've always feared. So naturally Xavier tells me it's just what I need.

Well, *he* might need it. But not me.

Problem is that since no one else is around to work on, I find myself wondering whether there isn't something in *me* I could change.

Some *small* thing. Which would actually be a pretty *big* change for me.

I realize that I've been looking for help and love and approval from others my whole life, believing that someone else could make everything all right. If I could only find the right man, he'd solve all my problems. Or, after I got sick, the right doctors. Now Xavier drones on and on about healing being a personal job. An inside job. I listen politely, but I still don't *hear* what he's saying. Because if it's true, I have nobody to blame but myself. And that's the one thing I'm not ready to consider. Let alone accept.

In other words I still don't get it.

Chapter Forty-Seven

In Hawaii, I see the head of family medicine at the hospital in Kailua every other week. We got to know him because he treated Liam's bout of hypertension. And after all, I need a local doctor in case my next illness-related emergency occurs on the island. To say nothing of routine blood panels and general check-ups.

I expect Xavier to disapprove. Instead he offers to go with me.

"You want to go to a *doctor's* appointment with me?" I ask, trying to figure what he's up to now.

"Change takes time," he says. "Besides, it's not us against them."

If it's not us against them, then what am I doing here?

I clear my throat in order to buy some time. "Are you saying you believe in Western medicine? That you think it can do me some good?"

"Of course it can," he says, as if surprised by the question.

Dr. B. turns out to be a breath of fresh air. He practices contemporary Western family medicine in a modern hospital, but he's also one of the most open-minded physicians I've ever met. Looks at the human body as a whole. Not as a system of separate components, only some of which are well.

Xavier sits in the exam room without saying a word, with the old half smile on his face. It's as if the doctor has his job to do, and Xavier has his job to do, but they don't have to compete for my attention.

Open-minded or not, this doctor isn't wild about the idea of my going off a few of my medications, and looks at Xavier as if this was his idea. But when Xavier explains that he's simply been asking me if I *feel* I can do without them, not telling me to stop taking them, Dr. B. reluctantly gives his consent. And for what it's worth, I'm sick and tired of swallowing pills and sticking myself with needles.

And there's something else too. A part of me wants to see if Xavier's right. That my body *can* learn to manage without the drugs. At least without some of them.

Chapter Forty-Eight

THE NEXT TIME he stops over on Oahu, Rob is sullen. I can tell he blames Xavier for the changes that are beginning to take place in me. Like questioning what my doctors tell me. Or what *he* tells me.

Father. Husband. Healer.

When a sick person starts to get well, those closest to her feel the consequences too. And on some subconscious level, they're not always prepared for their worlds to shift at the same time as that of the patient. Because for so long it's been about the sick person being sick.

And suddenly the sick person is well? Too big a change, thank you very much. We like things just the way they are. Broken.

And naturally Xavier has a story to make the point better than I ever could. "Did you ever hear the story about the bucket of crabs?" he asks me.

I shake my head no and try to act like I want to.

"Well, one day a woman walks down the beach and sees a fisherman. The fisherman's got a bait bucket filled with crabs, and the bucket doesn't have a lid. "'Aren't you worried that the crabs will get out?' the woman asks the fisherman, but he just smiles. 'Nope,' he says, shaking his head, 'not as long as all the crabs are in the same bucket. Now, if there were only one crab in the bucket, then yes, it would find a way out. But if the bucket's full, and one crab tries to escape, the others will pull it back in. That's just the nature of crabs. If they can't get out, nobody else is getting out either.'"

Chapter Forty-Nine

B Y THE FALL of 2007, both Cat and Cole were in high school. And it was around this time, after some irregular lab results, that an internist was able to rule out chronic leukemia. That was a big relief. But with so many health issues, it was always easy to imagine that something else would go wrong too. In the meantime, I continued to see my doctors and take my medications and to act like I had a life worth living. And to do what I could to offer my youngest kids a relatively normal life too.

An offer Liam and Nathan had already missed out on. In family therapy, Liam had finally admitted that my illnesses kept me from being the sort of mother I might have been. And Nathan added that I wasn't much of a disciplinarian either. He was right. It was hard for me to enforce the rules when I was so preoccupied with my own medical treatments. Which meant that our younger set got away with even more than the older set had.

Those days it seemed I was falling so fast that there was nothing to do but prepare myself for the impact. And try to prepare the kids too. It was around that time that all of us first grappled with how sick I really was, and what the end result would surely be.

So, with help from our family therapist I worked out what I wanted to say. "When I die," I told Cole and Catherine, "I won't really be gone. I need you to understand that. I will see you again. I will be waiting for you. Hold that in your hearts."

Chapter Fifty

I N THE LATE winter of 2011 my life begins to revolve around food. I spend obscene amounts of time in grocery stores, partly to shop and partly to ease the loneliness. Sometimes Xavier comes with me, and leads me around like a child, steering me past the cans and the jars and the boxes to the fresh fruits and vegetables.

"You have to change the way you think about food," he says, inspecting a bunch of Red Russian kale.

"I don't see why," I respond.

"Because you still think of food as nothing more than nourishment."

"You're right, I do. Especially since I can no longer eat a single thing I like."

He puts the kale back and turns to face me. "What I'm asking you to do is to try and think of eating and drinking as a way of *communicating* with your body."

"Okay," I say, "but I don't see the point. My body already *knows* I want a Diet Coke."

He ignores me and continues to look over the produce. Like a mother picking through clothes on sale, trying to find something her children will wear. "Communication involves listening, too," he says, sniffing some spinach. "It's not just about talking to your body."

"I am listening, but it's kind of hard to hear anything while my stomach's growling."

He shakes his head. "Of course it's growling. You've stopped dumping garbage into it, but haven't figured out what to put in its place."

"How *exactly* am I supposed to do that?" I ask him, bewildered by what he's asking me to do. And by all the choices in front of me, not one of which I want to eat.

"Just ask your body. It knows what it needs."

I'm beginning to think Rob's right. This guy really is crazy. What has Aliceanne gotten me into?

"And just as importantly," he goes on, as if I were hanging on his every word, "you need to use food to repair *trust*. To think of eating as a peace offering."

"No peace pipe?"

He inspects some Swiss chard. "What I'm saying is that your body needs to know you're going to take care of it before it can begin to heal."

He moves through the grocery store like no one I've ever shopped with. Picks things up. Touches them. Smells them. Puts them back if they don't seem right to him. It's a little weird to tell you the truth. But I'll say one thing for him, we don't tire ourselves out walking around. In fact, we avoid every part of the store but the produce section. And the aisle where they keep the bags of rice and beans.

"Just try to remember," he says, "that the same energy that grew these plants also beats our hearts. Breathes our oxygen."

"Okay," I say, "but what about the energy that grew a coffee bean? My body is *begging* me for a mocha."

"Stop resisting," he says, furrowing his brow. "There's nothing to be afraid of. Change is good. And it's not as hard as you make it out to be."

I want to believe him, but I'm tired. And hungry. "I don't know about that, but I do know how to listen to my body. In fact, I'm way

172

better at it than you think I am. And I can tell you with one hundred percent certainty that my stomach isn't growling because it wants a carrot."

"That's a victim's mentality," he says.

Which pisses me off so much that I storm out of the store and leave him standing there between the beets and the zucchini.

Chapter Fifty-One

IN APRIL 2008, Rob and I celebrated our twenty-fifth wedding anniversary, in California. Or rather, Rob insisted on celebrating it. If anyone had asked me, I'd have told them I'd rather stay home. I felt awful and I looked worse. And while my medical team was still doing their best to manage my symptoms, I wasn't getting any better. Everybody knew it. So celebrating anything, including what was left of our marriage, wasn't really at the top of my to-do list.

Especially because, by then I knew that I was going to pass the rest of my life in doctors' offices and hospitals. I knew that my husband was going to be on the road so often he might as well just move out. That my oldest son, Liam, was probably never coming home again. That his brother Nathan was far away in Colorado, and that his brother Cole was living in a haze. And although she was just a sophomore in high school, Cat was already a party animal and was always going to be a party animal. Her father's daughter, in other words. How many times had I awakened early and walked out into the living area to find her and her friends, and sometimes people even she didn't know, still going at it.

Celebrate?

Okay. It was true that Rob and I had gotten through twenty-five years together. And we'd had four beautiful kids. And had, thanks to Rob's hard work not just moved into, but had embraced the top income tax bracket. But I'd still rather have celebrated at home.

So of course Rob insisted on throwing a huge party at Fogarty's Winery.

Fogarty's is a Silicon Valley institution. It's only about fifteen minutes from our house on Westridge. From its site on the mountain Fogarty's looks down across Silicon Valley to the east, and toward the Pacific Ocean to the west. There are porches on all sides of the winery and both the food and wine are acknowledged to be some of Northern California's best.

Everyone who was anyone was at our grand anniversary party. By which I mean every one of Rob's colleagues. And his friends in the industry. Along with their gorgeous wives, wearing their expensive dresses. Me, I was draped in some gauzy, tent-inspired turquoise thing designed to hide my bulk. Probably made me look even bigger than I was.

After an hour or so I couldn't take it anymore. I slipped away to sit on a stone wall and look down at my swollen ankles.

Liam told me later he remembers that party as my worst moment. He was right. I weighed so much I felt like I was pregnant with all four of my kids at the same time. I had no energy. I was bloated and humpbacked by the steroids. And not an hour went by without my having to check my blood sugar or take one of my meds.

Eight years had passed since I was diagnosed with Addison's disease, and as the other diagnoses began to pile up my doctors hadn't lied to me. They'd told me my diseases couldn't be cured, only managed. They'd warned me that the treatments they prescribed would take their toll. And they'd certainly been right about that. The medications had systematically broken me down.

How long did I have to live? They couldn't say for sure back then. Only that with luck I'd be able to see all four of our children graduate from high school.

Which means that somebody ought to pull me off the shelf because I'm way past that expiration date now.

Chapter Fifty-Two

HEALING, XAVIER TELLS me, isn't just about changing my diet. Or giving up cigarettes.

There's something else, and that's what's keeping me from buying into Xavier's approach. I can't bring my family with me. I know that must sound silly, because a spiritual journey is obviously a highly personal matter. But Xavier still can't convince me that this shouldn't be a group project.

The family that transcends together finds peace together. Or however that old saying goes. Not that we necessarily have to *transcend*. I'll settle for something far more ho-hum, like say, a functional marriage, and four sober kids. But lately every step I take is accompanied not only by pain but by an unspoken fear.

By trying to get well in order to save my family, I'm afraid I'm going to lose them instead.

Chapter Fifty-Three

NATHAN CAME HOME the summer after the anniversary fiasco, just like he always did. He remembers driving me to and from doctors' offices the whole time. I was suffering from the first round of stress fractures to my feet. So I was in a walking cast most of the time. Or using a roll-about. Or worst of all, riding in an electric cart. If you've never had to, you can't imagine what it's like. You might as well wave a red flag and then beep the horn, just to be sure that *everybody* knows you're riding around in a cart because you're on the way out.

Below is an excerpt from my podiatrist's report that summer.

> Julie has a Jones type fracture, which are notorious for not healing. Given her history of immunosuppression because of dexamethasone use, I would recommend strict non-weight-bearing—which is standard for Jones type fracture—and a bone stimulator.
>
> . . . and Vicodin #30 to be used every six hours as needed for pain.

Another doctor. More medications. Even less mobility.

But it's funny how you look back on things. I have good memories of that summer, because Nathan would drive me to my appointments, and afterward he and I would go shopping for groceries. Or to Ross or Target. He'd unload my electric cart from the back of our SUV and off we'd go, doing our best to buy some momentary happiness.

And maybe it was that summer, I don't remember exactly, that for the first time I began to think we might all have been better off without the money. Without leaving North Carolina, where the kids and I were happiest. Without the riches that made all of this possible. By which I mean the house, and the cars, and the wine cellar. And the best health care plan in the solar system, as one of my husband's colleagues used to say. Covered every medication every doctor prescribed.

Chapter Fifty-Four

I'M MANAGING TO stay off bread and Diet Coke. Mostly. I'm still eating greens and lots of fresh fruit. But the dog bite still spooks me, and whenever I start to freak out, I dose myself with steroids, which is what Rob always told me to do whenever I was under stress.

"Just to be safe, dear."

It's a step backward, but my body is telling me that's what it wants. And Xavier is always telling me to listen to my body. There's just one small problem. My body's telling me one thing, while each of the *many* voices in my head is telling me another. And they're all squawking like mynah birds trying to make themselves heard. So which voice am I supposed to listen to? Which voice am I supposed to believe?

The next day I drive to Xavier's place for a treatment. Naturally I start by complaining. About having to listen to all the contradictory voices in my head.

"Your ego likes to keep you living in fear," he says. "That's how it stays in control."

To tell the truth, I'm beginning to miss the way the doctors always coddled me. To miss the belief that a pill, or even better ten pills, could cure my ills. To miss people telling me how brave I was. At least I knew who I was then.

I was the sick woman.

Now I feel like crawling out of my own skin. Like running as far and as fast as I can. But where am I going to go? I'm stuck. And as much as I enjoy my thrice-weekly treatments, I'm still tethered to my medications like a horse to a rail. I'm still a slave to the insulin pump and the steroids.

I had no idea how much work healing was going to be.

At least Xavier still believes. Without him I'd have quit a long time ago. So what does he do? He turns everything upside down and tells me that he's leaving.

Chapter Fifty-Five

NEAR THE END of 2008 fresh medical problems shoot up like desert flowers after rain. I see an ophthalmologist for flashes of light. They expand into circles and last for ten or fifteen minutes at a time. Typical of ocular migraines, the ophthalmologist tells me.

Worst of all is the incontinence. Such a sterile word. Doesn't begin to describe the humiliation of soiling yourself.

Okay. Babies don't care. And most mothers don't mind cleaning them up. For a few years anyway. But when you're in your late forties and your kids are grown and you wake up in the middle of the night and it's already too late to grope your way to the bathroom? Trust me, that's a whole different ballgame.

Just before the new year I go in for a routine visit with my endocrinologist.

Blood Pressure: 138/100
Pulse: 78
Weight: DECLINED

Yeah. You know you're in trouble when you decline to be weighed.

Chapter Fifty-Six

Xavier's leaving for Thailand to meditate and fast.

In darkness and in silence.

For twenty-two days.

At first I panic, but after a deep breath or two I'm able to ask him why.

"To elevate my frequencies."

"To elevate your *what*?"

"My frequencies. I do it every couple of years. If you raise your frequencies high enough they'll begin to vibrate with the essence of all things."

Is he kidding?

"So, let me get this straight," I say, choosing my words carefully, so I have a little more time to wrap my head around this. "You meditate, and you fast . . . in the dark."

"And in silence."

Of course. How else could you become one with everything?

He kneads my shoulders as he tells me this. "I don't always succeed, but that's my goal."

Sounds like some kind of transcendental boot camp. "But you're definitely coming back, right?" I ask him, one side of my face pressed against the treatment table.

He doesn't answer right away.

Is he already trying to raise his frequencies? While he gives me a massage?

"I also do it to keep from getting too comfortable," he says, ignoring my question. "Because the moment you get comfortable, you can no longer change."

"I don't know about anybody else," I mumble into the mat, "but I'd give just about anything to be comfortable again."

"That's because you don't see change as an opportunity."

He's wrong. I do see it as an opportunity. For a total physical and mental breakdown. Too bad he won't be here to see it.

I don't care what he says, I'm still not comfortable with the idea of being on my own. Especially not now. I've been looking over my shoulder at my old life more and more often. And I'm worried that, without Xavier around, I might just turn around and head for shore. Stop swimming toward something that's not on any map I know of, and start swimming back to what I know.

"I don't think I can make it on my own," I almost whisper. "I don't trust myself."

He snorts. "You're getting too used to being on my treatment table," he says. "And besides, you'll be surprised at how well you'll do. You've made a lot of progress. Just take care of your leg wound and use your juicer."

Again with the damned juicer. Which is still sitting on my counter, unused.

Okay. I feel guilty about letting it just sit there. Especially because it looks so lonely. But every time I think about using it there is suddenly, magically, something else to do. Like a load of laundry. Or floors to vacuum. Or bathroom tile that needs re-grouting. On some level I know that the juicer represents a threshold, a particularly significant step toward wellness. And once I step through that door it will slam shut behind me and there won't be any going back. But I don't want to lose that option. Not until I know what's on the other side.

And know that my family can come with me.

I see Xavier once more before he goes. He teaches me how to use moxa.

"What's *this* supposed to do?" I ask him.

"It's a form of heat treatment. It stimulates the circulation of Qi in the blood." In for a penny, in for a hundred bucks, I guess.

So now I'm supposed to hang little cones of mugwort incense on the insides of my ankles and the tops of my feet. Three times a day. And this is supposed to "untangle" my Qi along the kidney and liver meridians. And help support my adrenals. The healthy blood flow will also take the edge off any depression while he's gone.

According to Xavier.

Sure hope he's right. Because if it doesn't he's not going to be around to take the blame.

We do a trial run to make sure I know how to properly administer the moxa. That is, without giving myself third-degree burns. As I peel off the self-stick backing and press a light green-gray incense cone to one of my swollen ankles, I can't help being struck by the contrast between Xavier's "prescriptions," and those given to me by my Western doctors.

All the latter were either ingested or injected.

And there was no massage. Or acupuncture. Or focus on my diet.

In the six months or so that I've been working with Xavier he hasn't even prescribed any herbs. Instead he keeps steering me back to my relationship with my body. About the various ways to listen to it, to understand it. To care for it myself so that it can care for me.

This is so vastly different from what I experienced in the world of Western medicine that when I first started working with Xavier I almost felt cheated. My team of physicians, after all, *served* me. *They* checked my vitals. *They* drew my blood. *They* continually examined me, operated on me, treated me. I didn't have to do anything, other than put my health in the hands of the experts and silently follow their protocols.

Okay. Maybe not silently, but obediently.

It was them against my illnesses, and money was no object. I wasn't responsible for my own treatment or care. I was sort of a pampered observer.

I try to keep this impression to myself, but ultimately, I can't help pointing this out to Xavier. He laughs as he guides my hand to the appropriate spot on my right ankle to put the Moxa.

"Teach a girl to fish," he says.

Just before he goes, Xavier tells me again that this will be a good test for me. An opportunity to find out if anything I've learned has stuck.

"It's not a bad thing," he says. "In fact, it's a necessary part of making progress, of moving to the next level." And then he's gone, and I'm alone, again.

Chapter Fifty-Seven

OR THE FIRST few days after Xavier leaves for his retreat I lie in bed and stare at the ceiling. I *understand* what he said about this being an opportunity to move forward. But I've been at this long enough to know that it's also an opportunity for resistance. Resistance with its forked tongue and its gilded invitations. Encouraging you to return to the way things used to be. Promising that this time things will be *different*. That things will be *better*. If you'll just give it *one more chance*.

Xavier's words ring in my ears. "There are some tests we have to pass on our own."

Problem is I was never a very good student. I did just enough to get by. And I didn't particularly care for homework and practice, and I especially didn't care for tests. Once I was old enough to get out on my own, I preferred hanging out with boys.

Finally, one morning after Xavier's departure, I get out of bed and wander out onto the lanai and smoke a cigarette. I've given up smoking exactly the way I've given up drinking coffee. That is, I've given up *thinking* of myself as a smoker and a drinker of coffee. By the time I extinguish the cigarette, I'm already bored. Good thing my leg wound needs attention or I wouldn't have anything to do. So I take care of it as carefully as I can. I spend twice as much time as I need to. Then I check my insulin. Eat a bowl of oatmeal. Drink some tea.

Carefully burn some moxa. And by the time I finish it's still only 9:00 AM.

This is never going to work. I'm amazed by the way time expands when you find yourself alone. When you're around other people, it feels like there are only one or two free minutes in a day. When you're alone, there are a hundred empty hours. And this I think is a big part of my health problems. I don't know how to fill the time. I don't know what to *do* with myself.

I go back to bed, but I can't sleep. I get up and draw for a bit. Then, quickly tired of drawing, I read for an hour or so. Then swab my wound again and change the bandage. Fix a salad.

The clock seems to be moving in slow motion. It's not even noon, and yet I have completely run out of things to do, even though I've been doing things for an hour or two just to be doing something. Not because the things need doing. Or because they're particularly good for me.

Like more cups of coffee, and cigarettes.

My kids don't come over and they don't call. Rob is in Europe, I think. I want to pick up the phone and call one of them. But I just pick up the receiver and put it to my ear. I can almost hear their voices. Like hearing the ocean in a shell. But what would I say now, after kicking them out of the house? Xavier made me do it?

None of my options satisfy me. Everything is upside down. Why couldn't Xavier just sit in a dark closet here on Oahu?

Whenever a member of my Western medical team went on vacation someone else filled in. There was always someone to call. And there was always a hospital emergency room open somewhere. No matter the time. Day or night.

How can he call himself a healer if he takes off to care for himself? And leaves me to take care of myself?

It's cruel.

It's a violation of the Hippocratic oath.

Somehow I manage to keep resistance at arm's length, without

190

really knowing how I'm doing it. But I'm defenseless against depression and anxiety. My thoughts and feelings bump against each other like umbrellas on a crowded sidewalk in the rain.

I realize that my worst fear has finally been realized.

I am completely and totally alone.

Emotional malnutrition. That's what Eastern medicine considers Addison's disease to be. But that isn't Xavier's primary diagnosis. He says I suffer from an inability to love *myself*. More particularly, from an inability to *open* myself to love.

To receive it. Digest it. Absorb it into my system.

Which makes his the hardest of all my diagnoses to accept. Because considering the possibility that he's right makes me feel as if I'm drowning in a pool of my own tears. And if that's true, no wonder Western medicine can't help me. Injections and surgeries and pills won't keep my head above water.

And that turns the entire concept of health care upside down. At least as I know it. As I was trained to administer it. And that means I'm going to have to do the very last thing I wanted to do. The thing I've been avoiding my entire life. I'm going to have to take responsibility. And to do that I'm going to have to get used to being by myself.

Or as Xavier would say, being *with* myself. And learning to like it. By learning to love myself unconditionally.

"Only that," Xavier told me, "will allow you to heal."

In other words, I'm screwed. Because at the moment I can't even stand being in the same room with myself.

And yet somehow the days pass. I brood and cry and feed myself yogurt. Sometimes a bowl of ice cream. I know, it's not on the list. But if Xavier thinks he can just take off and leave me on my own, then I intend to take advantage of his absence. Decide for myself what I'm going to eat and drink.

And when I can't find anything else to eat that I *want* to eat, I stand in front of the refrigerator with the door open and stare at the insulin. Still hidden behind the open box of baking soda. Weirdly comforting to know it's still there.

Meanwhile I can't help but think of Xavier sitting in a dark room halfway around the world, offering himself to the energy that beats our hearts and breathes our breath. His mind free of ego. Seeking higher frequencies.

Maybe I'll drive into town and get a bacon cheeseburger and some fries and see if that cosmic ripple crosses the ocean and disturbs him while he's meditating in the dark.

Chapter Fifty-Eight

IN MARCH OF 2009 the associate professor of Clinical Medicine at the teaching hospital turned out another seven-page report. It was the last one I ever read. Actually it was the last one I could bring myself to read. It was an all too familiar roll call.

Addison's. Crohn's. GI bleeding. Diarrhea. Bronchiectasis. Chronic Sinusitis. Asthma. Colitis. Granulomas. Arthritis. Diabetes. Hypothyroidism. Prednisone. Enbrel. Humira. Remicade. Doxycycline. Biaxin. Imuran. Xifaxan.

I'm reproducing most of the seven-page report verbatim here as part of the medical record. And I won't blame you if you skim it. Or skip it entirely. It's just here in the book as part of the medical record. And for what it's worth, I can't bear to read it myself.

The patient was first seen at the IBD center back in 2002. At the time she was referred by a community gastroenterologist for management of suspected Crohn's disease.
... and there was clear evidence throughout the colon of a chronic active colitis with non-necrotizing granuloma seen [in] the cecum, transverse colon and sigmoid colon biopsies.
She was initially treated with medications such as mesala-

mine, with no impact on her constitutional or GI symptoms, because she was found to be Addisonian of unclear etiology.

From the year 2000 onward, she was managed with prednisone. This did have some positive effect on the GI symptoms.

She then developed arthritis, and was seen by a rheumatologist who started her on Enbrel for what was by his diagnosis a joint destructive arthritis, though apparently it was [sero] negative.

The patient then returned to the IBD Center in 2004, and came under my care.

I did not see the patient again until February 2006. In the interim, she underwent a laparoscopic Nissen fundoplication for reflux disease. She did receive Remicade, in an effort to provide her with a remission with respect to her destructive arthritis, as well as deal with the granulomatous inflammation of the bowel and her gastrointestinal symptoms, and in an effort to try to lower her corticosteroid use; though her Addison's would prevent probably complete withdrawal from corticosteroids.

She was hospitalized and underwent an extremely extensive workup by both Rheumatology, Pulmonary Medicine, Infectious Disease, and Endocrinology.

I saw the patient again in 2007. She came back now with progressive symptoms of abdominal pain, especially right upper quadrant pain, fatigue, malaise, low-grade fever, waxing and waning liver function tests, with transaminases as high as into the 200 to 300 range, and an elevation of alkaline phosphatase, and persistent and somewhat progressive additional gastrointestinal symptoms such as gas, bloating, and crampy abdominal pain and diarrhea.

I saw the patient again in April 2007, along with one of our hepatologists.

We sent the patient for CT enterography, which was normal without any clear evidence of gross inflammation of the bowel, anything to strongly suggest a diagnosis of typical Crohn's disease.

The patient was seen again [in the summer of 2007] by infectious disease physicians who failed to detect any infectious etiology for her symptoms, though she had clear persistence and progression of her symptoms. She was given additional empiric antibiotics including treatment trials with Levaquin, Fluconazole, and Augmentin, and we once again recommended a trial of Humira.

She had marked improvement in constitutional symptoms including resolution of fevers and chills, sweats, anorexia and weight loss. She had continued arthralgia of her joints, though this might have been somewhat better as well after initiation of Humira therapy.

With all of the steroid therapy, she had developed a chronic sinusitis, and in fact was even diagnosed with aspergillus in her sinuses. She was under the care of ENT physician, and apparently that infection was being controlled with the antifungal medication.

The last time I saw the patient in the office was in May 2008. At that time, she was having her persistent gastrointestinal symptoms with chronic loose stool, four to five bowel movements a day, the chronic vague abdominal discomfort, but no real major change in symptoms.

So my overall assessment is that Julie R. has a multisystem disease of uncertain etiology.

She clearly has a multitude of significant side effects because of the steroids, including chronic infections in the sinuses, bone abnormalities, and diabetes mellitus.

Chapter Fifty-Nine

ALONE MOST OF the day, I take to staring at myself in the mirror. I run my sausage-like fingers over my swollen face, allow them to rest on the black calico patches, gifts from the steroids. I strip down and stare at my naked body in the mirror, at my sagging breasts, at the hills and valleys of my stomach, my thighs. Trembling a little, I touch them, with fear and a little anger. Thinking back to all the ones who had made my body theirs. Or tried to.

My husband. My children as I carried them. My doctors. My first boyfriends. My cousin. The priest.

Standing there, looking at my body, with all its scars, visible and invisible, I see the story of my life. Is it possible, I ask, looking at myself in the mirror, that this body can still have a happy ending?

A couple of days later, I find myself standing at the kitchen counter in front of the juicer. I stare at it for a good long while. Finally, because I can't think of anything else to do, I make myself a juice with cucumbers, beets, and kale.

Chapter Sixty

B Y 2009 IT seemed like the bones in my feet fractured anew
every other month. It wasn't bad enough that I was sick, I was
breaking into pieces too.

And so was my family.

Rob had given up on me, and I don't think anyone blamed him.
The glory of his Addison's disease diagnosis was long gone. His heroic
support of his crazy wife was old news. By 2009, he was just stuck with
a chronically ill woman who was never going to get better. A woman
who hadn't even been healthy enough to care for their children while
he circled the globe, saving lives and making money. And finding
sexual release far from home.

In September of that year Cat and I got into such a vicious fight
that I had to go to the hospital for stitches in one ear. She pulled my
earring right through the lobe. She was seventeen, and she'd been
drinking.

Chapter Sixty-One

THE KEY TO juicers is to clean them as soon as you finish drinking your juice. At least that's what Xavier says. Or would say, if he were here. But like everybody else I know, he's somewhere I'm not.

I feel like I spend most of my time just cleaning the juicer. Not drinking juice. The machine seems to grow new parts overnight. And pulp from the fruit and vegetables somehow splatters into each and every one of those parts. Which then have to be scrubbed clean. It takes forever.

Xavier never seemed to care *what* I put into the juicer, although he did talk about how the juice of different vegetables does different things to you. Or for you. When he's around to talk, that is. Like cucumbers cooling you. Or beets raising your blood sugar. Or kale oxygenating cells because it has a lot of chlorophyll in it. Again, it doesn't matter to him as long as I juice three to four times a day. Which means that by the time I finally finish cleaning the damn thing, it's time to juice again.

But whenever I complained he always said the same thing. "How many pills do you take every day?"

I make vegetable juices mostly. Keeps my blood sugars from careening wildly out of control. I stuff spinach and carrots and tomatoes and celery and cucumbers into the chute. Then drive them into the spinning blades with the plunger. Kale. Collard greens.

Ginger thrown in for a little spice, and to minimize any residual gastrointestinal distress from the Crohn's. Fennel and turmeric to reduce inflammation.

Again, Xavier never seems to care what kind of juice anyone makes, just as long as they make the juice themselves. And since he's off taking care of himself, I'm thinking about tossing a pack of hot dogs and a few ice cream bars into the juicer. Maybe a liter of diet soda too, and a pack of cigarettes. I wonder what he'd say to that.

Probably nothing. That's his usual response whenever I challenge him.

But I know what he means. And I know he's right. The energy I put into buying the fruit and the vegetables, preparing them for the juicer, and then drinking the juice and cleaning the machine, delivers not only a steady stream of easily digestible nutrients, but also a daily lesson in self-nourishment and love.

"The easily digestible juices free up energy for cellular repair," Xavier always says, "and the process of making them is a lesson in unconditional self-love. In radical self-care."

Okay, but it still seems like *I* have to do everything.

Still, as I use a toothbrush to remove carrot pulp from the juicer's stainless-steel blades and basket, I begin to understand what he's talking about. It's about establishing a tentative sort of trust between myself and my body.

I'll take care of you. And stay out of your way. And you'll put me right.

It was also one more way to pass the time, without rehashing all the mistakes I'd made as a wife and mother. Or just hiding under the covers. And cleaning that juicer requires a great deal of focus, which forces me into the moment. And when I'm in the moment I don't hate myself. As much. Which isn't the same thing as saying I love myself unconditionally. Or even *like* myself. But it does seem that when I'm working with the juicer there's no time for self-loathing. No free fingers for pointing at anyone else either.

Chapter Sixty-Two

FEBRUARY 2011 TURNS to March and Xavier finally comes home. He looks freshly scrubbed. Lighter somehow. He can't stop smiling. Tickled, it seems, by what has been revealed to him.

"Life's just not what we think it is," he says. "It's so much more than the cramped little existence our ego-driven minds perceive." He tells me that once we see the truth of who and what we are, and allow ourselves to move beyond the restrictions conditional love imposes on us, we'll find that our daily lives can be almost orgasmic in their intensity.

I'm jealous. I haven't had an orgasm in years.

I have, however, been juicing every day. And cleaning my wound. And monitoring my insulin. So in some ways I, too, feel freshly scrubbed.

Okay, but I still lack any sense of peace. Or any real connection to the world around me. Still, I'm no longer swimming away from anything. Not that I'm swimming toward anything yet either. It's more like I'm treading water. Doing what I always did. Just going through the motions and keeping my head above water. And of course checking out of the corner of my eye to see if someone sees what a good girl I've been. To see if *anyone* notices.

Like Xavier.

At least this part of the process is familiar to me. In fact, I've become really good at it over the years. That is, at giving people exactly what they want. Good at being who *they* want me to be. Learning from a very young age to adapt myself to any situation. To earn praise. Or to blend into the shadows. I will do whatever I think you want. So you'll love me.

Or at the very least, not hurt me.

No matter how many times Xavier repeats the phrase, unconditional love is still just a cliché to me. I can't get my hands on it. Much less wrap my mind around it. Especially since the more I try to understand it, the less comprehensible it becomes.

Xavier tells me that's to be expected. "When we make a little progress, we all think we deserve a vacation. In other words, a return to our old habits, just for a while. Sometimes we even think that we've come so far that there's really no need to continue doing what we've been doing, to heal."

I like the sound of that.

But by now even I know that's the wrong answer.

One morning, a week or so after Xavier returns, I look into the mirror above the bathroom sink and see a lesion on my face. It's on the lower part of my left cheek, just above the jawline, about the size of a quarter. I go to my general practitioner, who sends me to a dermatologist. When she sees the lab work, she refers me to an oncologist.

"It's malignant," the oncologist tells me. "I recommend immediate surgery. It's our best option."

Our best option? Sounds more like *his* best option. To me it feels like a big step backward. Like an invitation to a reunion with Western medicine, where I'll see all my old friends. Friends I thought I'd outgrown, to tell you the truth.

And yet I'm not afraid. Which is unusual, to say the least. For decades I would never even have attempted such a measured response. At the time of all my previous diagnoses, or accidents, I'd always vacillated between total devastation on the one hand and superhuman emotional strength on the other. This time I simply step back, deciding that observation rather than engagement is the better way to go. Rather than feed the cancer with anxiety and fear, I'll simply let its energy move through me.

As for the inevitable intervention, I've been here before. I've sat in the waiting rooms, talked to the guys with white coats. Doctors with serious faces and serious voices. Tight smiles offered in vain attempts to inspire hope. Pre-ops and hospital gowns. Wires, tubes, and ice chips. IVs. Gurneys wheeled down fluorescent hallways. Bright lights. Scalpels. Eyes peeking out over blue masks. Then falling into the darkness of anesthesia.

"It feels like I'm betraying our work," I say.

Xavier smiles his crooked smile and shakes his head. "How many times do I have to tell you? We're not fighting Western medicine. Eastern healing and Western medicine can complement one another."

I start to say something, but he stops me by putting a fingertip on the lesion.

"There are no knives in Eastern healing, and this has to go."

Chapter Sixty-Three

IT TURNS OUT to be an outpatient procedure. They do the biopsy right there in the office, and it turns out to be a squamous cell carcinoma. So they just keep slicing pieces off, one after another, until the margins are clear.

The first thing I see upon regaining consciousness is a pair of kind eyes. As I get my bearings I see a nurse standing at my bedside. "Welcome back," she says, comforting me. "The surgery was a complete success. They got all of it, and the margins are clear. You're going to be fine."

Afterward, when Xavier comes to see me, he suggests that I stick to vegetable juices. "Cancer feeds on sugar, so no fruit juices for now."

No matter how comfortable Xavier is with the operation, and the way it went, it still feels like backsliding to me. Especially because, the week before, I'd gone three whole days without putting any insulin in my pump.

Three whole days.

I'd tested my blood sugar, just like I always did, but my levels were completely normal.

"Why're you so surprised?" Xavier asks me. "It's just your body's natural reaction to the respect you've been showing it. It's your body's way of telling you the changes are working."

Chapter Sixty-Four

A COUPLE OF WEEKS later I wake up early and shower. Get dressed and head into Honolulu. Feeling pretty good, I guess, without even realizing it. Maybe because I'm in a rush. Because I don't want to be late for my appointment at the spa.

When I get into town, I steer my car into an empty parking space. And then as I open my door I realize I forgot to attach my insulin pump this morning.

Shit.

I've also forgotten to pack my blood sugar monitor. And I was in such a rush that I even forgot to check my blood sugar before I left. A wave of anxiety sweeps over me.

Shit.

Still, my blood sugars haven't been fluctuating much, and I've needed less and less insulin over the past couple of weeks. But walking out of the house without even thinking about my insulin pump makes me feel irresponsible. Like one of those mothers who forgets her children in the store and doesn't realize her mistake until she's too far away to come up with any sort of reasonable excuse. I fumble around in my purse for my phone.

I'll call Rob.

No. I won't.

He'll never pick up. And even if he did, he'd tell me to go home.

Give myself some steroids *just in case*. And for reasons I can't really understand that would somehow feel like cheating.

Maybe I should call Xavier. But I already know what he'll say, too. "Quiet down," he'll tell me. "Listen to your body. Let it tell you what it needs."

Which is great advice, I guess, if you're asking your body if it's hungry. And if it is, whether it feels like sautéed spinach or cheese curls. But blood sugars are a little different. If I don't hear what my body is telling me about them, I could be in real trouble.

Further complicating the situation is the fact that a diabetic's mental faculties deteriorate when blood sugars fluctuate too far from the mean. Which doesn't sound *so* bad unless you're a nurse and you know that the next phase could be a coma. So while I feel fine and think my mind is clear I know my condition can shift on a dime.

I close my eyes and draw in a deep breath. Curl my fingers into a fist, so I can't press my panic button. Sit, at rest, and listen.

My heart beats like a hummingbird's.

Not really at rest, but all right. Just a little strange. A little, dare I say it.

Normal?

Can't be. I draw in another breath. Exhale slowly. And then like a hunting dog raise my nose to the wind and sniff.

Nothing.

I open my eyes and look around the parking lot. Maybe I could ask a passerby if *she* thinks I should keep my appointment at the spa. I could just head straight home. Or better still, go right to the emergency room. But of course no one walks by, and eventually I realize that I'm going to have to trust myself this time.

So I make a bold decision. I get out of the car and walk toward the building. Telling myself that I can check my blood sugar when I get home. At the moment I just don't feel like I need any insulin. And for the first time in a long time I'm confident enough to take a chance.

But of course *my* voice isn't the only one in my head.

"Well," interjects a high strung, nagging voice I know so well, "I hope this little experiment doesn't cost you your life."

When I get home, several hours later, I rush inside to check my blood sugar.

It's 98.

Totally normal.

I breathe in deeply, then exhale a slow sigh of relief. Decide I'm going to put the insulin pump next to my pillow so I don't make the same mistake again tomorrow morning. But when I check my blood sugar the following morning the numbers are still normal. I never put the pump on again.

Chapter Sixty-Five

BY THE SPRING of 2011, my family is in open revolt. I have diabetes but no longer wear my insulin pump.

"Are you crazy, Mom?"

"Do you have some kind of a death wish?"

"Who does this weirdo think he is anyway, telling you to stop taking your meds?"

I've heard it all before.

If a team of the best doctors in the Western world couldn't cure me, what makes Xavier think *he* can? No way to explain to them, really. Xavier's not telling me to do anything. Except listen to my body.

My kids aren't the only ones questioning Xavier's influence.

Francesca is a beautiful French-Portuguese woman I've known for years. She's probably just about as free a spirit as you can be and still keep your feet on the ground. She has a head of wildly curly salt-and-pepper hair that spills down her back like a waterfall and a belly laugh that radiates outward like ripples in a pond.

Maybe she was a gypsy in a former life.

In this life, however, she is a massage therapist. She comes to my house once a week to give me deep tissue and Hawaiian lomilomi massages. "Xavier is too harsh," she tells me. "Too masculine."

What can I say? He *is* masculine. But *too* masculine?

"Men think *their* way is the only way," she continues.

"Oh come on," I respond. "Xavier would never say that."

Her laugh is like a flash of light in a dark place. "No, but he *thinks* it," she said, still smiling. She begins to knead out the tension in my lower back.

How does she know what Xavier's thinking? Besides, even if it's true, maybe that's what I need. Someone strong enough to push me. Not some pushover.

"And who can blame him?" she went on, her hands gently probing. "We've always accepted men's power over us. We don't question it. So they just keep telling us what to do."

My doctors maybe. But not Xavier.

"Unless," she goes on, "*we* say no."

I'm tired. And the massage is making me sleepy. But I know that at least part of what she's saying is true. Xavier has joined the line of powerful men in my life. Or maybe, as Francesca says, the line of men to whom I've *given* power.

A line that extends from my father.

Through my husband.

And now to my healer.

"He pushes you too hard," says Francesca.

"I know, I know," I say with a sigh. "But the thing is, I've got some really fierce resistance to change, so it takes a lot of force . . ."

". . . change can't be forced," she says, interrupting me. "Even Xavier will tell you that."

That spring Francesca and I travel to Maui together to study Reiki healing. On the way back from Hana, she jerks the wheel to the right until the car skids to a stop on the side of the road. Then she bounds out of it like an animal.

Before I know it she's out of her shirt and bra. And the next thing I know, she's dancing topless under a small waterfall.

I wade carefully into the sparkling pool fed by the falling water.

214

With my shirt still on. Standing there, waist deep in the pool, I watch Francesca as she bobs in and out of the waterfall, her face split by a sparkling grin. She raises her arms toward the heavens, and her laughter echoes off the rocks. Wraps its arms around me.

My hands fall to the hem of my shirt. I twist my fingers into the fabric. Try to summon the daredevil in me.

But I can't do it.

So I just stand there and watch her instead. Marveling at her spirit and wondering what sort of breakthrough it would take for *me* to finally be able to unlock myself and dance topless in a Hawaiian waterfall.

Chapter Sixty-Six

THERE WAS NEVER any plan.

Getting off insulin just happened. It wasn't an act of courage. It just came from buying into the process. Otherwise I'd never have risked it.

Makes me think of taking the kids to the pediatrician for their childhood immunizations. The doctor would say the same thing every time. "Okay, on the count of three. One . . . two . . ."

And then he'd stick them with the needle *before* he got to three. Because when we know something painful is coming we instinctively clench our muscles, and that makes it even harder for the needle to go in. Which makes the experience that much more painful.

If I had known my body no longer needed the insulin I probably would have tensed up. Been frightened by the change.

"It's hard for us to let go," says Xavier. "Hard for all of us. We're so attached to the identities that our egos have constructed for us, and that the societies we live in have approved. But these false selves . . . mother, daughter, wife, sister, sick person, victim . . . they disappear once we see them for what they are."

He's got that part right. I do feel like a lot of my old selves are disappearing. And it's about time. But not taking my insulin still scares the shit out of me. At the same time I'm beginning to feel things moving inside me. Things that have calcified over the years and are now coming back to life.

Xavier tells me it's all good. "This is a natural result of the new relationship developing between your body, your spirit, and your soul," he says. "Just stop trying so hard. Nurture yourself instead, like you would a newborn."

I don't want to be a newborn again. And I definitely don't want to learn how *not* to try. I want to do something. Help the process along. Do my part. I want to put my shoulder into it. It's what I've always done.

"And that's what's kept you from healing," says Xavier, sounding a bit exasperated. "There's nothing for *you* to do. The process of healing isn't yours to take charge of. Or mine, for that matter."

"But I have to do something or I'm gonna go crazy."

"So, go make some juice. Take a walk. Go shopping. Burn some moxa. Just understand that it's arrogant to think *you* have the ability to heal yourself."

That hurts. I'd never once thought that participating in my own healing would make me *arrogant*. I'm just trying to helping myself.

"The way you talk about it," I tell him, "I feel like I'm back in a hospital, lying in bed while the nurses and the doctors do everything."

He shakes his head.

"Do you see any doctors or nurses around here?" he asks, sweeping one arm around to take in his treatment room. "No one is directing your healing here. Not even you. I'm just trying to help you get out of your own way."

In other words, every time I find a new purpose in life someone tells me to stop. Maybe Francesca's right. I'm a nurse. And I've spent ten years going in and out doctors' offices and hospitals trying to manage my own care. And now all I'm supposed to do is just sit around and love myself unconditionally? Oh yeah. And keep juicing. And quit smoking. And live alone and survive on seeds and beans and roots and fruits and vegetables.

I don't know. To me living like a monk seems just as arrogant as believing that I can heal myself.

When I get home I decide to monitor my vitals. Before I know it, I've got numbers spread out in front of me like some college student cramming for a math exam. I begin to email Xavier with updates every fifteen minutes.

> Blood sugar up to 180. Added steroids. Blood sugars dropped to 110. Now the question becomes do I add insulin instead of steroids? I just slept for 15 hours. Maybe for just a short time increase steroids a small amount and let things settle?

Xavier is as patient as ever. "The key here is *knowing* that you're pushing too hard," he says. "Stop struggling to prove to yourself that you don't need the medications. Just keep ingesting a steady stream of . . ."

". . . I know, I know, easily digestible, natural nutrients."

"That's right, and let your body decide what you do and don't need. Reduced dosages will come as organically as you forgetting your insulin pump. Just stop competing. It's not a fight."

Still seems too simple to me. For years and years I've worked as the head nurse for the only patient on the floor.

Me.

Always vigilant. Always as disciplined as I could be. Aware of everything that went on and everything that was going to go on. Now I'm being told to retire. To ignore the doctors' orders and let the patient direct her own care.

How does that old line about a lawyer representing himself go?

Oh yeah.

He has a fool for a client.

Chapter Sixty-Seven

WHENEVER I'M FEELING really lost I draw. Probably just some sort of Obsessive Compulsive Disorder.

Xavier disagrees. "Drawing is a form of meditation, just like running, or playing an instrument, or cooking. Or best of all, gardening."

For him maybe. I've got two black thumbs. But I can draw, so I know that what we see, and what we *think* we see, are rarely the same thing. In fact, we never actually *see* what's in front of us. Instead, we see our *perception* of what's there. A reality created by filtering visual data through preconceived ideas and preexisting emotions. Then, depending on what we *want* to see, our brains add and subtract inputs, making what we see more attractive. Or repulsive.

Xavier, as always, knows how to sum that up in a sentence.

"You can't look at what you're drawing," he says, "when you're looking at what you're drawing."

I'm finally starting to understand why I've always been so terrified of being alone. Why I'm still terrified of being alone. It's all about perception. Of what I saw as real when I was a child.

I was extremely close to my paternal grandmother, my father's Hungarian mother. I loved going over to her house. Especially when hostilities broke out at our place, which happened pretty often.

But knowing that my grandmother's house was a sort of refuge for me, my parents often punished me by forbidding me to go there. They sent me to my room instead. And somewhere along the line I began to associate being alone with punishment. A perception that continued and intensified throughout my marriage. One after another, Rob's career moves ensured that he and I would spend less and less time together. Leaving me alone. Punished. But without knowing what I'd done wrong.

I came to this conclusion, strangely enough, through the process of drawing. And suddenly, I found myself less afraid of being alone. Maybe it would have happened anyway, and just occurred coincidentally while I was drawing. Doesn't really matter, I guess.

"There is a wonderful story in the Zen tradition," Xavier says one afternoon as I lie on his treatment table. "A professor goes to visit a Zen master. The professor chatters on and on about wanting to learn the teachings of Zen, the traditions of Zen, in short, anything and everything there is to know about Zen. Meanwhile, the Zen master quietly pours his visitor a cup of tea. As the professor talks, the Zen master keeps pouring. Eventually, the cup becomes full, but since the professor continues to talk the Zen master continues to pour. Finally, the tea overflows the cup.

"'Stop pouring,' the professor cries out. 'No more will go in!'

"With a smile," says Xavier, smiling himself, "the Zen master gently tips the teapot back and sets it down.

"'This is you,' says the Zen master to the professor, indicating the brimming cup. 'Already full of your own opinions and speculations. How can I give you anything else unless you first empty your cup?'"

Chapter Sixty-Eight

"THE TIME IS coming to ask your body if it really needs the steroids anymore," says Xavier, the next time I see him. "To ask your body if it's able to make what it needs on its own, just like it did before."

This is still such an overwhelming idea that I don't know what to say.

"Remember, you *accepted* their treatment," says Xavier. "No one held a gun to your head. So you can *decline* their treatment too."

"Easy for you to say. You're not the one who has to go cold turkey."

"No, I'm not, but you had to have known that this moment was coming. And surely you didn't expect your body to just shrug off the side effects all at once."

I say nothing.

He strokes his Fu Manchu meditatively. "Maybe it will help if you think about the way you take your winter clothes off, layer by layer. Finally, it's spring, and you find you don't need any of them anymore."

"Okay, but it's not my fault. They're the ones who say I have to wear this stuff all the time. They're the reason I'm so used to being overdressed . . ."

". . . assigning blame is a dead-end street," he says, "not a path forward. But if it's true that these guys overdressed you, then they *ought* to have to watch you while you strip back down."

"Let's try going a week or two without Trilipix," says Dr. B. during my next visit. Xavier's there, too, simply looking on. "Especially since you've got diabetes *and* hypothyroidism," Dr. B. continues. "And to tell you the truth, I don't know why they put you on it in the first place."

On the way home Xavier suggests I ask my body about nicotine, too. "Ask your body if cigarettes should go the way of Trilipix," he says.

"I quit smoking a long time ago," I lie to him.

"No, you didn't," he responds, but without making it sound like an accusation. "And I think your body will tell you that the time *has* come because the cigarettes are part of the reason your body isn't producing its own steroids."

Chapter Sixty-Nine

R OB IS FLYING in from Geneva. And because I'm feeling better I look forward to seeing him. Yet a few hours after he arrives, his presence begins to irritate me. Is it him, or have I somehow gotten used to living alone?

It makes sense. Our lives have veered off in different directions as my diagnoses piled up, to say nothing of years and years of escalating treatments. And his constant traveling. But we still lived in the same house, still went through the motions of being married, of being parents to the same children. Of staying together, 'til death did us part.

Don't forget, Julie, I'm Catholic, and Catholics don't believe in divorce.

Now, after six months of working with Xavier, it seems as if health, not death, is beginning to come between us.

I try to share my progress with him anyway. He listens politely. But I can tell he isn't really interested. For him it's enough to know that I'm feeling better. That I'm not going to be making any additional demands on his time. No need for the details. And he is equally uninterested in reevaluating the treatments I'd received over the years.

"You had some of the best doctors in the world . . ."

". . . and what good did that do me?"

He looked up at the ceiling. "I'm not going to get dragged back into this. The labs don't lie . . ."

". . . I know, Rob. I'm a nurse, remember? And I know the labs don't lie. But that doesn't mean that *treating* disease is the only approach. There's something to be said for searching for the root cause, too."

It might not sound like it, but I still want to keep my marriage together. I want it badly. But when my husband's around, it seems like all my hard-won energy drains right out of me.

Thirty years of marriage and four children. Now it seems like we're looking at each other from across the room. Pretending we're still together. Or *acting* like we're still together. Like me healing was what we *both* wanted. Now I'm not so sure.

By the end of the first day I know. And he knows, too. Even if he doesn't say anything.

We can't live in the same space anymore. Not if I want to continue to heal. Which means I'm going to have to focus on myself for now. Figure out how to fit back into my marriage later. And my family. If there's anything left to fit into.

The healthier I get the farther Rob seems to float away. Or maybe I'm the one floating away. Either way, I can't play at being his wife anymore. And even though my illnesses have been hard on my children, I have to get well.

Because that's the only way I'll ever be able to take care of them again.

And Xavier says *that's* the real problem. Of course.

Chapter Seventy

I AM EIGHT MONTHS into the healing process. I've eliminated two of my daily medications. And just as Xavier predicted, my daily dosage of synthetic steroids is falling. Maybe one day my body won't need the thyroid meds either.

Dr. B. is amazed. "How have you managed to heal so rapidly?" he says, staring at the labs and shaking his head. I shrug my shoulders.

I don't know what to tell him. Except to repeat what Xavier always tells me. "Given the right conditions, as long as there hasn't been any irremediable damage, the body will eventually heal itself."

My doctors prefer to consider it a miracle. An outlier. Or at least an unexpected and inexplicable remission. Which does happen. As a nurse I've seen it myself. But it really comes down to this, for the doctors, it's better to chalk it up to a miracle than to a simple, natural process they can't or won't understand. To do that, they'd have to admit that they were more interested in the diagnoses than they were in looking for the *cause* of my illnesses. To say nothing of the wild idea that their treatments might have actually done me harm.

First do no harm.

So they prefer to call it a miracle.

Okay. Maybe not all of them. Dr. B. is definitely open to an alternative explanation, some kind of unknown cause. But then again he saw my progress with his own two eyes. And for those who didn't, my *miracle* sounds so simple it's almost embarrassing to talk about.

"Um, yeah. So, I almost died, but then I drank a lot of unprocessed juice, and ate nothing but whole foods, and got a bunch of massages and acupuncture treatments. Oh, yeah. And I told myself 'I love you a lot.'"

Xavier says that the most important thing I did was exit the downward spiral of my life. Step out of the whirlwind. He says that my healing began the moment I left my entourage of doctors and my melodramatic life in California. I don't know if that's true or not. But it really doesn't matter. What matters to me is that as I heal, I also have reason to panic.

I'm going to have to face the fact that healing will reveal me for who I really am. Which is the last person I want anyone to see. Not after all those years of wearing my autoimmune diseases the way some women wear make-up. To cover up their blemishes. And their insecurities too.

I was just a skinny little girl who wanted to be loved. A little girl who thought it was her fault that she *wasn't* loved. Who thought it was her fault that her family was such a mess. Who thought it was her responsibility to save *them*.

And a little girl who had failed. Twice. First with the family she was born into and then with the family she and her husband had created.

Of course I *still* want to heal. And of course I'm thrilled to finally be able to look into a mirror again without looking away in disgust and shame. I still weigh more than a hundred and fifty pounds, but that's way below my high. I've even bought some new clothes. Just the same, without the cover of my illnesses I feel like I'm walking around naked. I'm not sure what people might see without my illnesses covering me.

Despair? Shame? Fear? Self-loathing?

"That's just your ego talking," says Xavier. He sounds as tired of making the point as I am of hearing it. "Can't you see," he continues, "that this is just fresh evidence of your addiction to drama?"

"That is *so* not true," I say, knowing perfectly well it is.

So what do I do? What else? I get a tattoo.

Okay, in retrospect maybe not the smartest choice I could make at the time, given my suppressed immune system. But it's not fancy or large. In fact it's just one word.

HOPE.

Written in blue-black ink, in the lacy script of the islands. Chosen because faith and trust seemed like such long shots. But Hope? That I could do. And now, every time I walk along the beach, I look down at my right foot and remember.

To hope.

Chapter Seventy-One

"HAVE YOU THOUGHT about meditation?" Xavier asks me, as he massages my feet. "It might help your body move to the next level of wellness."

Caught off guard, I don't know what to say.

I've changed my diet. I've stopped smoking. I've gotten massage and acupuncture treatments two or three times a week for the better part of a year. And now I'm supposed to start meditating? Me, who can't stand being alone? Shutting myself up in my mind?

"There's an ocean of difference between health and wholeness," he says. "Physical health is the body operating at maximum capacity. Every cell vibrating with energy, in rhythm with every other cell."

I would kill for a cigarette right now.

"Wholeness, instead, is a trinity of wellness," he continues. "To be whole your physiological, psychological, and spiritual systems not only need to work well individually, they need to work harmoniously. If there is disease in one, it affects the other two."

Three systems? Wholeness? What happened to juice and acupuncture? To just getting healthy?

"Thanks," I tell him, "but I think I'll just stick with the health thing for the time being."

"When we are whole," he goes on as if he hadn't heard a word I'd said, "we are aligned with the essence of all things, and are one

231

with the divine. And when we are one with the divine, disease cannot exist."

I want very badly to keep my mouth shut, but just can't let it go. "So, are you telling me that if I can become one with the divine I can go back to smoking cigarettes?"

"Of course not. What I'm telling you is that meditation will allow you to find your way into the quietest recesses of yourself. To the places where true transformation can take place. Where the different parts of you finally begin to cooperate."

I shake my head almost imperceptibly. "It's never gonna happen. I can't even stand to be alone in a room. Forget about being alone in my own mind."

"Stop resisting," he says. You're at war with yourself, and you have been all these years. That's why you got sick, and it's why you can't heal."

Maybe, but meditation still scares me. Because I know that if I clear my mind, I'll have to face the truth that being sick worked for me. "Okay, I admit I've been hiding behind my illnesses. But I still don't see why I have to learn to meditate . . ."

". . . would you *stop* creating more drama?" says Xavier. "Meditation is just an opportunity to love yourself more completely. To love even those parts of yourself you fear, that you've pushed into the darkness so you don't have to face them."

"Well, what if I don't want to look at all my failed selves?"

His hands move to one of my calves, massaging it until the tension is gone. "Refusing to face yourself is no way to go through life. Besides, it's keeping you from becoming whole. It's blocking divine energy, so it can't course through you. Can't cleanse you. Can't *energize* you."

Okay. He had me there. I *was* still tired. Not as often as I used to be, but still too often.

"Well, can I take a few days to think it over?"

He looks at me closely. "After all this time, and after all the progress you've made, you still can't commit?"

My mind scrambles, searching for a way out. "I thought meditation was about openness and light," I say, "not about confession. You know, parting the veils so you can touch the divine."

"That's one part of meditation," he responds, working his thumbs up my spine. "But before we go up we must go down, and as we descend, our false selves abandon us."

"I'd kind of like the company for now, if it's all right with you."

I can't see him, but I *know* he's shaking his head.

"Trying to achieve wholeness is the ultimate test of your commitment. To achieve wholeness, you have to abandon everything you believe about yourself. Everything you cherish. You have to tune out all the old, worn-out lies, and meditation will help you do it."

"That sounds like a lot of fun," I say, "but I can't even sit on the floor, much less cross my legs."

"Not today, maybe. But you'll be able to one day. In the meantime, you can begin by trying to be mindful."

"Could we just stick with the massage? I'm tired of thinking."

"Being mindful isn't the same thing as being thoughtful. I'm talking about being mindful of your food as you eat it. Feeling its texture on your tongue and lips. Being mindful of the hands that grew it, cared for it, and made it available to you."

"Look. How about a break? For just a minute? My head is spinning."

After he finishes my massage, we head toward the beach. Once we get there we walk along in silence for a while, and then Xavier asks me another question, out of nowhere. "Did you see the flowers on the shoes of the woman we just passed?"

"Nope."

"Did you notice how many birds were playing in that puddle we just walked by?"

"Of course not. But I get it. You're telling me that I can't be mindful of flowers on shoes or birds in puddles when I'm so caught up in my own thoughts. But who cares about flowers on shoes or birds in puddles?"

"The point is to calibrate your eyes and ears, so they can follow the yes."

"So they can 'follow the yes'?"

"Yes, so they can follow the yes."

I don't really get it, but I try to be mindful just the same. No matter where I am. In the grocery store I play the observer. Pay particular attention to colors and designs on boxes of pasta. Or on cans of soup. I run my finger down lists of ingredients, stopping at the ones I don't recognize, and then asking my body if it would like some. And then I listen very carefully.

Or I try to anyway.

"Essence always offers us guidance," Xavier tells me, "but we have to learn to see it. Learn to hear it. Over time, you'll even begin to feel it in your body."

He can tell I'm not getting it and smiles.

"Try this, then. Tell yourself, 'water is good for my essence.'"

"Water is good for . . ."

". . . no, no, not out loud, say it to yourself. Then be mindful of how your body responds to the statement. Be mindful of what it feels."

He waits until he figures I've had enough time to give it a try and then continues. "Now tell yourself, 'Cigarettes are good for my essence,' and listen again."

Like he doesn't know how that one's going to turn out. "That," he says, after giving me a little more time, "is how you calibrate the 'yes.'"

A couple days go by before I see him again, but Xavier starts right in as if our previous conversation had never ended.

"Mindfulness is what separates the sages from us. Being mindful, they are always prepared to follow the 'yes.' In fact, they follow it as a matter of course. Without question. Even when essence seems to point them in an illogical direction, or one in which they do not wish to go."

I understand this instinctively since I was taught very early on not to trust my inner voice *or* to follow my inner compass. I learned instead to be guided by the opinions and needs of others.

Parents.

Teachers.

Ministers.

Or put it another way, I was taught to look outside myself, not inside myself, for the one true direction.

I give it my best, but calibrating the 'yes' isn't nearly as easy as Xavier makes it out to be. Especially since the answers to most questions aren't as clear-cut as they are for water or cigarettes. And sometimes, although I'm sure Xavier would deny it, there seem to be differences of opinion within essence.

Or even indifference.

When, for instance, I ask essence if whole-wheat pasta is good for my body, essence seems to shrug its shoulders. But if I ask it whether or not peanut butter cookies are good for my body, an argument breaks out between two different voices. And just like old times, I'm left to play the peacemaker.

Too much sugar and processed ingredients, one side argues.

Yes, but we like peanut butter cookies, the other side fires back.

Before five minutes have gone by, I'm so dizzy that I walk right out of the store. Leave my cart right in the middle of the cookie aisle. Okay. Maybe the cookie aisle wasn't the best place to start. But I thought I'd give myself a real test. Not just stand in front of the kale and ask a question I already know the answer to.

"Don't be so hard on yourself," Xavier tells me. "It will come."

But I can't help myself. I always was and still am obsessed with getting things right. Even if I know it's a process, and that I can't succeed unless I allow the process to take place. Mistakes and all. That said, I can only imagine the beatings I'd have gotten if I'd tried to pull something like this when I was growing up.

A few days later I walk the aisles of the supermarket again. I don't really need anything. I'm just there to calibrate the 'yes.' So why do I feel a knot of anxiety in my chest? I stop in front of a display of rice crackers. Ask my body if it would like some for lunch, then listen for an answer. But my body must be in the middle of something because it doesn't answer. So I bear down. Breathe in and out, like Xavier's taught me. Try to shut out the cries of the toddler in a shopping cart at the end of the aisle.

Sounds like his mother won't give him something he wants.

235

There's a burst of static from the store loudspeakers. Then a surreal voice announces the specials of the day.

Please tell me that's not the voice of essence.

It's not easy, but I finally shut the store manager's voice out too.

Focus my eyes on one box of crackers.

Listen only to myself. And in a snap of the fingers the answer comes. Although I don't really hear a voice. I just feel it. But the message is clear.

If it comes in a package, you don't need it.

Chapter Seventy-Two

XAVIER ENCOURAGES ME to keep seeing Dr. B. He also encourages me to work with other healers.

"Anything you do out of love for yourself will help you heal," he says, inserting acupuncture needles into my skin. "Especially if you can do so while keeping in mind that at bottom we are *energetic* beings. Every single cell in our bodies is energized by the flow of essence. And we monitor that flow through the seven chakras," he adds, resting one palm at the base of my spine. "From the root chakra to the crown chakra, which sits, aptly enough, on the crown of the head."

Finally an image I can embrace. "So that makes me a queen, right?"

He chuckles. "A drama queen, maybe. Now quit fooling around and focus on your breathing." He waits patiently, saying nothing until he feels me relax.

"Like I've told you before, the chakras run along the vertical midline of the body. For some people, it's helpful to think of them as a connection between heaven and earth, as a sort of conduit for divine energy. When our chakras are open, which is their natural state, energy flows freely through us and we experience well-being. When the chakras become blocked, problems arise. These blockages usually occur as the result of us holding on to negative thoughts. And emotions like anger, resentment, disappointment, guilt, heartbreak, abuse . . ."

"... slow down, would you?" I tell him. "How am I going to remember all of this?"

He laughs out loud. "You don't need to write them all down. Besides, they're not the only things that cause blockages. Hanging on to any emotion is damaging to your system, because by its very nature energy prefers to remain in motion. So clinging to the memory of a first kiss, or satisfaction after a long-hoped-for promotion, can also create blockages."

"Great. They get you coming and going."

He laughs again. "Yes, they do. Even beautiful stones block moving water."

Chapter Seventy-Three

I FLIP THE CALENDAR to July. Almost ten months have gone by since I started working with Xavier, and Rob decides to fly out to the island and throw a Fourth of July party. Which is about the last thing *I* want to do. But he insists.

"It's a chance to bring the family together," he says.

The family I'd left behind in California and locked out on Oahu. Sure to be a festive occasion. We hadn't all been in the same room since Christmas.

When Buddha bit me.

More good memories.

And *that* wound took six months to heal.

"You know, it looks like an Omega symbol to me," says Xavier, inspecting the scar as he kneads my calf.

An Omega symbol? Isn't that the last letter of the Greek alphabet? So, does that mean I'm at the end?

The tide is out the afternoon of Rob's party, and a powerboat shuttles our guests to and from the sandbar that emerges only at low tide in the middle of Kaneohe Bay. From our patio it appears as if our guests are walking on water.

Rob is certainly in his element here. Still as handsome and as charming as the day I met him. There are tables everywhere covered with food. And ice-filled coolers with bottles of water and soda and beer and white wine. And just like the shuttle boat to the sandbar, they're all props in the play.

After all, people are watching. And Rob has a reputation to uphold.

I've lost a lot of weight. I look and feel healthier every day. And I think that's why Rob wanted to throw a party. In fact, I know it is. So *his* guests will be shocked by my transformation.

I feel like I'm on display. A sideshow freak outside Rob's Big Top. He wraps one arm around my shoulders and kisses me on the cheek. I smile and thank our guests for their kind words. And start to shrivel inside.

Rob and the kids stick around for a few days after the party. And once again the house is filled with drama. Drinking to excess. Heated arguments. Same shit, different day. I want to ask them to leave. To give me back my space. But the words stick in my throat.

Didn't I want to get better so I could care for my family?

Well, yes, I did. At first. But I'll never get better this way. And neither will they.

Rob tells me he's begun to look at me again. In fact he thinks he might even want to *sleep* with me again. You know. Now that my body isn't so grotesque.

I stare at him. Try not to cry.

It's as if I'm seeing him for the first time, as he really is. The guy I'm married to. Had children with. But who still doesn't see *me*. Or if he does, he sees only my body. Attractive to him again.

I reach for the steroids.

Worse still, I turn my anger inward. The way I always did. Which is what got me sick. Or at least contributed to the severity of my illnesses.

That night I lie in bed and stare at the ceiling. All that work for nothing. What an idiot I've been. To think that if I got well things could be good again between me and Rob. As soon as my family sobers up, they'll all leave again. Rob will fly off to his other life. The kids will go back to their lives.

And I'll be alone. Again.

But for the first time, after months of working with Xavier, I kind of like the sound of that. Actually, I feel like I *need* some time alone. For some quiet reflection.

But of course the moment they're gone I miss the chaos.

I call Xavier. "It just doesn't seem fair," I tell him. "Why do I have to *choose* one or the other. Can't I have both?"

Xavier is silent for a moment. "What did you think was going to happen as you healed?" he asks me.

"I don't know," I say. "I guess I thought that since I was getting better, they'd get better too."

Another silence. "It doesn't work that way, Julie. I can't do your healing for you, and you can't do their healing for them."

So it was me or them. Just what I'd always feared.

"Why don't you just let it go?" he says. "Start living in the present, because that's all there is. Everything else is an illusion."

"My children are not an illusion, and if you had kids you'd know that."

Another short silence.

"Of course your children aren't an illusion. And neither is your husband. But for years and years you've wasted your energy trying to create the illusion that you're all part of one big happy family. And now you're angry because you still prefer that illusion to reality."

Then he hangs up.

His words hit me like perfectly weighted punches, and once again I fall into a bottomless depression.

Nights are the worst. I lie awake thinking.

If only I'd been good enough. Strong enough. Smart enough. Then I could have saved them all. My parents. My siblings. My husband. My children.

241

Myself.

Which means that Xavier was right. There's never been any point in blaming somebody else. *I'm* the problem, and always have been. And knowing that hurts far more than being sick *ever* did.

I call Xavier back and tell him what I'm feeling. "You're exactly right," says Xavier. "You *were* the problem. But now you're the solution."

Part V
Returning

Chapter Seventy-Four

THE FOURTH OF July party really rattled me. It actually came close to derailing my healing. But I won't bother you with the details. The important thing is that after a few weeks, the clouds of depression dissipate, and I emerge into the patchy emotional sunlight feeling a bit battered. But still glad to feel the warmth. To find myself on my feet. So, I take a deep breath and begin my regimen of self-care all over again. And before long I'm back into my routine. Yoga and juicing. Massage and acupuncture. Occasionally some Qigong and moxa. A little lomilomi.

Aches and pains still sneak up on me from time to time. Mostly joint and abdominal pains. The last remnants, maybe, of sickness and disease rising out of my subconscious. There's no denying that the process is a sad one. But just like Xavier said it would, the sadness dissipates and the pain floats off into the sky. If I can just let it go. Only then will I receive the gifts of joy, peace, and unconditional love.

"When the last lie falls away, you'll meet your true self for the first time," says Xavier. "And you'll be warmed by the light of love, and overcome by the sensation of joy."

I sure hope he's right. Because right now those words sound a lot like a bumper sticker on a car that's almost out of gas.

Weeks pass. I continue to reframe my life. To see it as it really is. From a healthier and more loving perspective.

Whenever the kids show up, I try to stay strong. I'm now able to see how heavy a burden my illnesses have been to our children. All those years spent worrying that I would be hospitalized, or die, while Rob was out of town. Back then, fear hung over all our lives like a dark cloud. The experience forced me to stay awake at night, obsessively monitoring my blood sugars and steroids so I'd be alive in the morning. So my kids wouldn't have to fend for themselves.

But now I realize that was a big part of the problem. I think back to a family therapy session Cat and I attended together years ago, during which she broke down and lashed out at me. She, too, was afraid I'd die. But she was afraid that if I died, *she'd* be the only woman left to care for her father and her brothers.

"Because to me that's what it means to be a woman," she said. "You have to give yourself away. You have to live for men, never for yourself."

The knowledge that this was what I had taught my only daughter about womanhood settled in my bones like cancer. And she'd been only thirteen years old at the time. How many more ugly memories has she stored away?

And what about the boys? What must it have been like for any of them in the years leading up to my Addison's diagnosis? When on some days, the best I could do was just curl up in a nest of blankets on my bed.

I take a deep breath. Then slowly release it. Then breathe in again. Should I go to the gym? But either essence doesn't hear me, or it can't be bothered.

Which is just as well. After visiting the gym I almost always feel like crying. There are so many beautiful young women in there, it's hard not to think back to a time when I was as young and as beautiful as they are now. Back when Rob used to look at me the way young men in the gym look at these young women.

Ah, well. Guess the time has come to consider the beauty of the spirit. Something no mirror can reflect.

Chapter Seventy-Five

"**Y**OU PERSIST," SAYS Xavier, "in trying to see the things you *want* to see. Instead of being grateful that you're beginning to be able to see things as they truly are."

Things as they truly are. Who can remember? Especially because my memories of the last year aren't linear. They're kaleidoscopic, continually spinning around one another. Their colors and shapes shatter like colored glass, only to reassemble themselves in dizzyingly new forms.

I want to smoke a cigarette, lie in bed all day and eat ice cream. And of course, feel a little sorry for myself. But I don't. Instead I force myself to go to the gym. And then I go shopping, and when I get home I cook myself a good meal. And then I take Be out for a walk on the beach. Spend some time alone with the universe, as my dog races along the shifting line between the ocean and the land.

I don't always find peace.

And while sometimes nothing seems to make sense, I have decided that I'm no longer going to use my limited energy to walk *away* from the wreckage of my past. I'm going to start walking *toward* my future.

"Good for you," says Xavier, the next time we see each other. "But don't force it."

So I just continue to work at it. Steadily. As patiently as I can. Even if sometimes I know I'm just going through the motions. Still not really *believing* that my body can heal this way. Has healed this way, cleansed itself of incurable disease with the energy of self-love.

Then I make a really big mistake. I email Rob.

I thank him for being my teacher, and let him know that I have learned a lot from him. But I also point out that the lessons have been costly. So I won't be continuing my studies.

Okay. So it's a little dramatic, but old habits die hard.

Secretly I hope he'll write and tell me how proud he is of me, how beautiful he thinks I still am. How much he still loves me. How much our marriage and me and our children still mean to him.

He doesn't reply.

At the very least I hope we can still be friends. Hope we can salvage *something* from our long marriage. It's the only way I can think of that we can re-purpose our relationship, not lose each other entirely. As it is now, I still waste entire days thinking about him. About us. My thoughts and emotions swing like a pendulum, wanting him and not wanting him. Trying to pull him close and then pushing him away.

"Concentrate on your own healing," says Xavier.

Chapter Seventy-Six

I'M FEELING A little manic-depressive. Or bipolar. Or whatever they call it these days. One minute I'm on a rocket to the moon. The next I feel like I've stepped off a cliff.

"After more than ten years on synthetic steroids, of course you're going to have some wicked highs and lows," says Xavier. "You're just going to have to ride them out."

My ears hear what he's saying, but my body's not getting it. It's like my right foot is dancing to one tune and my left foot to another. One thing's for sure, if I sit around here any longer being tormented by my thoughts, I'm going to go crazy.

I decide to reserve a week in a yoga center on the Big Island. Just reaching for the phone makes me feel better. A little yoga and a change of scenery are just what I need.

The phone rings, and then an answering machine picks up.

The center is closed.

I feel like I'm following the "no" today.

I want to go back to bed. Pull the covers over my head. But I don't. And somehow just because I *tried* to do something, I feel a little better. So instead of lying down in defeat I make some green tea. Which makes me feel even better. And then something Aliceanne always used to say pops into my head. "You can make plans," she'd say, "but you can't keep them from changing."

So what, I ask myself as I sip my tea, is the point of making plans?

251

I call Xavier. For the twentieth time in the last eight hours.

"I'm so restless," I tell him, "I'm going crazy."

"Relax," he says. "It's just energy finding its way through you again, and it's a good sign. It means you're getting ready to move into a new realm of wellness."

"Great," I say. "Can I start packing?"

I can almost hear him rolling his eyes on the other end of the line. "Why do you keep trying so hard?" he asks me. "Don't you want to get well?"

This has *got* to be a trick question. I mean, how can I get well if I don't try? "So, let me see if I've got this right," I say, trying to sound as snotty as I can. "To get well I have to stop trying to get well?"

"You know exactly what I'm talking about," he says. "So stop complicating things. Stop setting up schedules. Just feed yourself, drink plenty of juice, stay active, and most importantly, stay out of your own way."

"But I still don't understand how . . ."

". . . you don't *need* to understand anything. All you have to do is believe in your body's ability to heal itself."

But I do *need* to understand. That's just how I am. And I'd also like to know how much longer this is all going to take. There *is* an endpoint isn't there? I mean the rest of my life isn't going to feel like this is it?

Sensing how fragile I am, Xavier does something that genuinely shocks me. He comes to my house to give me a treatment. "I didn't know you made house calls," I say. "I could have saved a lot of gas over the last year."

"Ssh," he says, putting acupuncture needles in my ears. I close my eyes and breathe into my heart.

"In *Zen in the Art of Archery*," Xavier continues, now inserting needles into the tops of my feet, "the master asks his student to observe a bamboo leaf in a snowstorm. As the snow accumulates, the leaf bends ever lower, not resisting, simply accepting the weight, until finally it bends so far that the snow slips effortlessly to the ground."

He pushes needles into the insides of my wrists. "The point is that the leaf itself does nothing," he says, "and as a result, it is not exhausted by the effort."

I hear what he says. But If I don't do something I'm going to go crazy.

Chapter Seventy-Seven

"You know, you could come by every once in a while," I tell Cat when she finally answers her cell.

"You're the one who moved out," she responds, "not me."

Okay, she's right. But it's not like I ran off with the tennis pro.

Nathan is in California with Rob. It seems in fact as if each member of my family is spinning off in his or her own direction. And without so much as a backward glance.

I haven't heard from Rob for four days now.

For the first decade of our married life we saw each other every day. And even after we moved to North Carolina and he began to travel, we still spoke to each other every day. And I mean *every* day.

Okay, it was over the phone. But we still spoke.

Sometimes we'd be separated by so many time zones that his voice seemed like a radio transmission from a distant planet. Reaching me long after the planet itself had ceased to exist.

You're being a nuisance, I tell myself after another phone call goes directly to his voicemail. You're getting needy again. He's out there living his life. While you're here living yours. And making a lot of juice. And after everything you've been through and everything you've learned, you're still sitting here wondering if he cares about you. And worrying not only that wherever he is, he's with someone else, but that he's been with other women for years. Decades even.

Six days go by, and still no word.

A week ago he flew to South Africa to accept an award for his research on AIDS vaccinations. Cole and Nathan went with him. I knew when I heard about it that it would be a good trip for them, but I still can't help feeling abandoned. As though they're choosing him over me.

All I ever did was get sick. I wasn't a bad mother. I just didn't have the energy.

An hour or so later I convince myself that Cole and Nathan's absence is a good thing. It really is. All right, I'm not *totally* convinced. But at least I'm able to *act* like I'm convinced. Even though there's no audience in the room. That's got to be worth something.

With my newfound perspective, I realize that I need these moments of peace more than I need their company. That the boys, too, need some space to adjust to the changes we've all gone through. This way no one's tripping anyone else up. Besides, I tell myself, I'm much more productive alone.

And I almost believe it.

The afternoon passes very slowly. It's amazing how much time frees up when you don't have to spend almost every waking moment treating your illnesses. I know I need to do something. Not just sit around and think. I need to do something important. Maybe choose color patterns for the kitchen. That might do it.

Rob finally responds to my email.

I hope you get well so someday you will be able to travel with me.

Travel with *you*? Why can't *you* spend a little more time at home? Maybe if you had, I wouldn't have gotten sick. I email him back.

call if you want to

Hoping I sound nonchalant about it.

Another day passes without a reply. So I give up on nonchalance and call him. But of course I can't reach him in South Africa. So I wait.

And wait.

And wait.

Which is what I've been doing my entire life, isn't it? Waiting. But now, finally, I find myself wondering just what on earth I'm waiting for.

Finally, he calls. He sounds rushed. It's clearly no more than an obligatory call. And realizing that makes me even angrier than waiting did. "I've had enough, Rob," I say. "Enough of these hurried phone calls. Enough of the quick visits that just disrupt my life and my routines. Enough dinner parties for people I don't care about."

It's as if someone else is speaking. Because what *I* want to say is that I love him, that I miss him, that I still believe in us and hope he feels the same way. But that's not what comes out. "I'm not going to live according to your rules anymore."

For the first time in my life I really feel schizophrenic. Angry.

Then compassionate.

I know it's always been hard for him to express his feelings. Maybe he's doing the best he can. God, listen to me, would you? Doing the best he can? I sound like a post-war housewife. The truth is, he's running away. That's what he's really doing. And maintaining the pretense that he does it to support our family.

Of course to be fair, I've done my share of running, too. I took my wedding band off two years ago. And he never even asked why. Or maybe he didn't notice. I rub the skin on my finger where I used to wear the ring. I draw air into my lungs, embarrassed by how I've been unable to smother my anger during our phone call. Who knows when I'll hear from him again? I didn't want to make him uncomfortable. Push him farther away.

Tears well up in my eyes as we wish each other good night, and then he hangs up the phone.

When Rob started to travel, and for the first time in our married life I couldn't reach out and touch him, I would build elaborate fantasies about how things were going to be. One day. This was just a temporary inconvenience. And luckily for me, I couldn't just sit around twiddling my thumbs. I had four children to raise, and a house to keep up. So I convinced myself that with enough positive energy I could still have the marriage and the family I'd always wished for.

One day.

Wrong again.

When Rob flies in from South Africa on his next visit, he looks at me the way he used to. Or something like the way he used to. He tells me I'm looking more like my old self. That he wants to touch me again. Make love to me.

These are words I've been waiting to hear for ten years. But now that he's back, there's nothing I want more than for him to be gone.

Maybe I am finally going crazy. I mean, I know how this must sound. And I'm not proud of it. Because I really *do* miss him when he's gone. But as soon as he re-enters my space I can feel myself beginning to orbit him. Like a planet in the gravitational pull of the sun.

But I do want to go to bed with him.

And then I don't.

I feel as if I need my meds. But I don't give in to that mad impulse. I do, however, give in to Rob.

Afterward I feel cheap. I feel used. Angry with myself. Not with him. Angry that I let him breach my boundaries so easily. Angry because I was unable to say no. Angry for not being able to care for myself when my husband is around in the way I can when he isn't.

258

Chapter Seventy-Eight

AWARE THAT ANGER has begun to block my chakras, as Xavier would say, I tell Rob that I'm thinking about enrolling in the School of Oriental Medicine in downtown Honolulu. I've even started filling out some of the paperwork. "That's a good idea," he says, surprising me. "Now that you're feeling better, it'll give you something to do."

It's the careless cruelty of this comment that stuns me.

I want to shout out loud that healing still gives me plenty to do. Doesn't he have *any* idea what I've been through? And then realizing that I am once again allowing my anger to obstruct my energy, I focus on settling myself. Draw in a deep breath.

Just whining. That's all it is. Not who I really am, just a habit it's going to take a while to break.

We drive downtown to check out the school. While there, we discuss the possibility of me renting an apartment near the campus. So I can walk to my classes.

"Well, if you want to rent an apartment, we're going to have to sell one of the houses."

Another casual statement that knocks the air out of me. Because I know he's talking about selling one of the houses on the island. Not the California property *he* lives in. The Hawaii property *I* live in. And it's a statement. Not a question.

To be fair, we *had* talked about renting the yellow house once

I got better. Which makes sense, I guess. But this is different. Now he's talking about *selling*. And there's something about the *way* he tells me that makes me feel like I'm sick again. Like I'm invisible. A patient in a hospital room somewhere. Not the woman he's sharing his life with.

How could I have fooled myself into thinking that we were moving in the same direction?

And then, in the moment that follows, I find myself wondering if this is the first move of his plan to leave me. Is that it? It kind of rings true. Especially if there's someone else. Is that what he really wants? To leave me and go to someone else? And if it is, can I go on without him? Can I continue healing, continue taking care of myself, without the idea of us getting back together?

I'm not sure I can.

Chapter Seventy-Nine

"I DON'T THINK I can do this anymore," I tell Xavier over the phone.

"Why is that?"

"Because no matter how much I do, it'll never be enough." I hear a bird squawking in the background, and for a moment I wonder if that's what *I* sound like.

"What happened this time?" he asks me, his voice steady, like that of a parent attempting to calm an emotional child. So I tell him about my last conversation with Rob. Or at least I try to tell him. Between sobs.

"Look," I say, after finally catching my breath, "I just can't do this anymore. Not by myself. Not just for me. I can't."

He doesn't respond.

Did he just hang up on me?

Then I hear him draw a deep breath in through his nose. "You are the only person you *can* do this for," he says patiently. "But you have to stop looking outside yourself. You need to look within."

Maybe. But looking inside myself is a dangerous business. Especially when I'm feeling a little off physically, which could be the result of my body reacting to my poor emotional state. Either way, that morning I awaken feeling a little feverish. Cole is in California, so I call Cat and asked her to check in on me later in the day. At the time it doesn't seem like a lot to ask.

But of course she never calls.

And then Aliceanne's ghostly words come back to me. "Rob and your children aren't doing anything wrong, darling. They're just living the lives they want to live, so don't waste your time blaming them. Start by looking at yourself. You need to start taking responsibility for your life."

God. Do I really have to learn this lesson over and over and over again? Aliceanne made that point years ago. And now Xavier makes it almost every time I talk to him. "Sit with yourself," he says. "*Allow* yourself to be lonely, and then learn to find your way around the loneliness. Learn to navigate it, not to be afraid of it."

Easy to say.

I almost spit the next words into the phone, unable to control myself. "Why is it so wrong," I ask, "to want someone I gave birth to, and cared for, to love me?"

"Good," says Xavier. "You're angry." Once again he's turned the tables on me.

"But I don't *want* to be angry anymore."

"So, let your anger out, and listen to what it has to teach you."

Then he says he has to go. Another client has just arrived.

For the next hour, I sit on the patio fuming. I'm angry. Like I should be. The way any woman who had dedicated the bulk of her life to people who don't seem to give a shit about her would be. I mean, is asking my daughter to call, just to make sure I'm all right, really too much to ask?

Guess so.

My anger rises up like a swarm of hornets. Self-care is out of the question. I can't even summon the strength to make a cup of tea. And for the first time in months I think about the vials of insulin in the refrigerator.

Are they still there? And the moment that thought enters my mind I'm ashamed of myself. One more incident with a selfish kid? *That's* enough to ruin a year's hard work? I'm not that weak, am I?

No, I'm not. And I know it. So I just breathe. Actually, it's not that easy. I have to *force* myself to concentrate on my breathing, and as I do the last few sane brain cells in my head tell me to call Xavier. Tell me it's okay to ask for help. So I do.

Xavier says he'll be at my place within the hour.

As I wait, I half expect Xavier to be angry with *me* when he gets here. To chastise me for playing the drama queen, when I should be making peace with reality. But he doesn't. He just asks me to lie down. To find my way to the center of the pain and to be with it.

Silently.

As his hands work on me.

When he's finished he tells me I can sit up, and when I do he puts a book about chakras into my hands. I know he's just trying to distract me. But I still appreciate the effort.

"Reading this," he says, "will remind you that you are more than your pain. It will remind you that you are made of divine energy, and that allowing that energy to move through you freely is the only way to heal."

I am made of the same energy that breathes my breath and beats my heart. That grows the plants in the pots on my porch. That guides birds on their migratory paths. The same energy that calls the humpbacks back to their birthing grounds off the coast of Maui.

"If you let it," he tells me, "that energy will guide you, whenever you're lost, and don't know where to go."

Finally, he reminds me, in addition to death and taxes, there is one more certainty in life. And that's change.

"Change," he says, "is at the very heart of life. So stop clinging. Let divine energy pass through you. Let it change your course. Change you. Allow alchemy to occur."

Chapter Eighty

A s I leaf through the pages, Xavier continues to talk to me. To console me. "Blockages in the first chakra are connected to adrenal diseases like Addison's. Blockages in the third chakra," he says, "which controls personal power and self-esteem, are connected to diseases like Crohn's and diabetes."

I raise my head and give him a grim smile. "Are you sure there are enough chakras in here to cover *all* of my illnesses?"

He looks at me without expression. "The throat chakra," he continues, pointing to the next page, "governs truth and personal integrity. So it gets gummed up by things like suppressed feelings and unspoken emotions."

I begin to read that paragraph. It says that when we fail to speak the truth we actually choke ourselves. Sometimes even to the point of death. And I realize as I read this that the throat chakra and the thyroid are found in exactly the same place in the human body.

Before long I'm not on the page. I'm *in* it. And as I read on, one simple, warm, revealing message radiates out of the book, like heat from an incandescent light bulb. I alone am responsible for keeping these channels open. I alone am responsible for my health and well-being. I cannot blame my parents. Or my husband. Or my children. Or my doctors.

Why has it taken me so long to understand this? It couldn't be simpler. I guess because it was always so much easier to blame someone else, rather than take responsibility. Besides, when you begin to point the finger where exactly do you stop? With your parents? Your grandparents? How far back does blame reach? Does it extend to the first human? The first living being? The first cell?

I guess the point is that once blaming others begins, it never ends. The cycle will continue until *someone* finds the courage to break it.

By the time I finally look up from the book I'm a little dazed, but at peace. And alone.

Xavier left without even saying goodbye. Or maybe he did, and I didn't hear him.

I draw air into the deepest recesses of my strengthening lungs and look around the room. Alone again. But for some reason it doesn't bother me as much as it did earlier.

Chapter Eighty-One

IT GOES ON like this for another month or so. I have good days and bad days, jerked back and forth between euphoric hope and suicidal despair. My steroid needs fluctuate wildly. When I feel like I'm suffering some sort of physical crisis they're the first thing I think of. But having learned a little about following the "yes," I am usually able to pause. In other words, no automatic responses. Not anymore. Ask, and then listen. Western medicine or Eastern? Food or steroids? Meditation or a cigarette?

"This is killing me," I tell Xavier over the phone.

"No, it's not," he says, without the slightest emotion. Like he was doing something else that was really important and listening to me with just one ear. "You're just going through the final stages of withdrawal."

Withdrawal?

"I don't know what you're talking about . . ."

". . . yes you do, and you saying you don't just proves my point. Did you really think that after taking all those drugs, for all those years, you'd just be able to stop whenever you wanted to? Without any side effects at all?"

"I don't know," I say. "I never really thought about it . . ."

". . . probably because you didn't believe you could do it. Just like you didn't believe you could climb that hill. But you *are* healing now, and a big part of the process is letting your body know that it's time get back to work. That you're no longer going to feed it things it can make for itself. And naturally, that's going to piss your body off. Doctors call it withdrawal."

I keep asking my body for answers, but some days all I get back is static. So like every good drug addict, I default to the steroids. And feel relieved and guilty at the same time. Because from time to time my body has *hinted* that it may no longer need the steroids. That I may be able to produce cortisol on my own again. In fact I've even been feeling a dull aching in my lower back. As though my adrenals were trying to kick-start themselves.

Xavier, as usual, cautions me to go slowly. "All change requires adjustment," he says. "Your body is just beginning to find its way again. While it does, nourish yourself, be still, and be patient. And when you have doubts, don't harbor them. Let them move through you, and leave you."

Rob emails me. Says he'll call. But he doesn't. Three days have gone by since we last spoke, and as embarrassed as I am to admit it, I find myself sitting by the phone like an insecure teenager. I force myself to get up, to walk around. Try to do something, anything. And when that doesn't work, I sit down and *will* the phone to ring. But of course it doesn't.

Is this me? Or me wanting the drugs I used to give myself.

Cat stops by. I can tell she's angry with me again, but she won't say why. Liam is mad at me too. I don't blame them. I'm still all over the place. And the pace of change has been so rapid, over such a relatively short amount of time, that all they're all watching me become someone they don't recognize.

Things would probably have been different with my children if I'd been better at setting boundaries, instead of thinking of my own childhood and trying to do the opposite. The truth is that I enabled them from the day they were born, taught them their mother would sacrifice herself for them. Taught them and their father that it didn't matter how they treated me. That it was okay to use me, to walk all over me.

Before I met Xavier, I thought unconditional love meant denying your loved ones nothing. It's what I was taught as a child. If I say "yes" to you, and give you what you want, and do what *you* want me to do, I'll earn your love.

I try to stay busy so my mind won't have time to turn on itself. Otherwise I'll lose control. And perspective. Not be able to hear the "yes."

I've made it clear to Rob that I don't want to sell this house. And to make the point even clearer I decide to redecorate. After all, it's *my* house. My plan is to make the yellow house *my* space. Just for me. And as I do, I realize that in all the years I worked to make our California houses into homes, I never once stood back to admire my work. I was always so focused on making sure everyone else was comfortable that I never enjoyed the fruit of my own labors.

When I run out of things to do inside the yellow house, I begin to tend my patio garden. A few months earlier Xavier and I had spent an hour or so on the lanai, planting rosemary, thyme, basil and lavender. Okay, we had to plant everything in pots, but Xavier said it didn't matter. It would do me good anyway.

"You need to learn to care for other life-forms without smothering them, and plants are a good place to start. Gardening also shows us the effect positive thoughts have on biological systems, including our own."

Then, when I was ready to go, Xavier handed one of the flats to me.

"Now, if *they* live, *you* live."

Just what I need. Something else to worry about.

But the plants do keep me busy, and I do a lot of drawing, too. I also lose myself in classes at the School of Oriental Medicine in Honolulu. Fill my mind with ancient wisdom about medicine wheels. About Qi. About pressure points.

And for reasons I don't understand, I also steadily increase my steroid usage.

"Just be patient with yourself," says Xavier. "Did you think you'd just wake up one morning and be healed? That you'd just stop taking the drugs you've been taking for years without taking a few steps back?"

He's right of course, and so I don't let it get to me. I just try to keep busy. And it feels good to be busy. Stressful but good. Moving is way better than sitting still. Even if I don't always move forward.

I write papers and read books. Take tests. I smile a little more. Sleep a little better.

And then I hit my biggest emotional challenge yet.

Chapter Eighty-Two

I**T STARTS OUT** innocently enough. Rob wants to take a trip back east to visit family. My family. I'm still in school, but since I've dropped one course, my class load will be manageable. That said, I don't really want to go. I'm not feeling up to it physically or emotionally. And I haven't really traveled since I settled in Hawaii in the fall of 2010.

Trying to maintain your distance from the first environment in which you got sick is a tricky thing. How do you explain to your family of origin that in order for you to continue to heal, you have to stay away from them? It's not a matter of blame. It's more like what an addict is told when he or she emerges from rehab. Stay away from the people who helped you become an addict. So the question is, can I stay well out in the "real" world?

The trip starts out okay. I see my sister and my brother, and cousins I haven't seen in years. Some of them are excited by how much I've healed. Others are uneasy about the way I've done it.

But I'm not the center of attention. My dad is really sick and my mother sticks to him like glue. So, flush with my own success, I try to explain to him that healing and health are an inside job. That we have to own our illnesses first, and then take personal responsibility for getting well.

He pats my hand. "Just be a good girl, Julie, and make Rob happy."

Rob doesn't need my help being happy, because my whole family fawns over him as usual. The rich good-looking doctor. How did I get so lucky? And they all talk to him, not to me, about how *I've* gotten well. If I try to talk to them about Xavier and the things I've learned about emotional malnutrition their eyes glaze over. And then Rob jumps in to tell everyone about his latest trip. Or a promising research project.

By the second day of the trip I feel invisible again.

It all wrenches me back to a different family gathering in Hawaii. Rob's family this time. Only a couple of months back.

We were all sitting out on the lanai of the yellow house. Me, Rob, his sister, Madeline, and her partner, Stacy. Stacy is a physician, too, but unlike Rob, she's changed her practice to incorporate holistic approaches to healing. In part, I hope, because of what she knows about my experience. She'd recently changed her diet too, and so had Rob's sister, and as a result they'd been able to reduce their blood pressure medications. They were clearly proud of themselves, and they said they were proud of me too.

Rob took a sip of his wine. "Julie may be all right now," he said, "but she'll be back on her medications sooner or later."

Rob's sister gave him a look. "Why would you say that?"

Rob looked her in the eye, then glanced at me. "Because I know her. She can't live without her meds. Not for long. Just watch."

I felt as if I'd been punched in the gut. I tried to stop the tears from welling, but I couldn't, so I just looked away, unable to imagine why my husband would say such a hurtful thing. Of course, it wasn't like that was the first time. I can't even count the times he's told me he wasn't responsible for my illnesses. All the times he's reminded me that I was damaged long before he met me. How he always told our children that my illnesses weren't their responsibility either. They just needed to live their lives, he told them. Let your mother worry about hers.

Which brings to mind the endless international vacations he took with the kids. A safari in Africa. The major cities of South America. They'd leave me at home because I was too sick to travel. And whenever I'd ask if we could take a family vacation closer to home, Rob's response was always the same. "Are you really so selfish that you'd deny your children these experiences?"

When he put it like that, it *did* sound selfish. So year after year I watched them pack their suitcases and head for Rome or Tokyo or Rio de Janeiro, while I stayed behind.

A new picture of Rob begins to emerge from this patchwork of memories. Like a slowly emerging Polaroid. Did I marry an abuser?

It sounds so awful. Even when you just say it to yourself.

To be fair, Rob never hit me. Unlike my father. So there were never any bruises you could see. But what is marginalizing me over the years if not abuse? And did he do it because of my illnesses, or were my illnesses the result of him doing it? At least partly.

Worst of all is what it means if this is true. If, after trying so hard to avoid recreating the circumstances of my childhood, I have to face the fact that I have actually perpetuated the ugliness I grew up with. That I'd just given my children another variation on the childhood I'd gone through.

On that trip to Maryland, for the first time in my married life, I begin to look at Rob as if I'd been partially blind over the past thirty years. Like I'd known my husband only by running my hands over his handsome face, by feeling the warmth of his body. In the safety of the environment I believed we'd created. But without ever *seeing* him or our marriage for what they really are.

And knowing that everyone else still sees Rob as the golden boy and me as the crazy one doesn't make it any easier.

The trip continues. And yet this time, for the first time, as I feel myself being drawn back into old routines, my *body* resists. As if now *I* am no longer blocking its path and *it* wishes to go in a different direction. A healthier direction.

But it's such hard work, and I begin to wonder why I'm fighting these battles here. Now. Yes, I'm getting better, but I'm still not in a position to devote valuable energy to fighting off attacks I could just as well avoid. I want that energy to be available for healing, because I've still got a lot of healing to do.

For the rest of the trip I feel as if I've got two enormous dogs on leashes, each one pulling me in a different direction. One represents the life the people I love are leading. This life they still expect me to lead. The other the life is the one I know I have to lead in order to heal. Put another way, I no longer want to expend the energy to listen to the "no," instead of the "yes."

In the last few days of the trip, I visit the scenes of my childhood, my parents' bedroom, the attic that I played in. We even visit my grandmother's house with the blue wallpaper. Maybe trying to remember who I was before the abuse began. Before I accepted their belief that I wasn't good enough to be loved. Or before I started to believe that that's what they thought. Before I got sick.

I think I was trying to say good-bye. I had to let go of the little girl and the young woman I'd been, in order to fully embrace the woman I was becoming.

By the time we return to Hawaii I feel as if I'm going to have to start from scratch again. Rob leaves for California, tells me he's had enough of my "whining." So have I. But for the first time in my life, I'm happy to be on my own again.

Chapter Eighty-Three

NATURALLY, THE FEELING doesn't last. One step forward and two steps back.

As I approach my fiftieth birthday darkness seems to settle over me. Not physical darkness. Not the absence of light. The darkness I encounter when I look inward, and another thick fog of depression settles over me again.

And yet I begin to see that if I stop struggling and allow depression to pull me into its dark core, I'll find myself in a womb of sorts. A place of safety, with the time and space in which to grow. A lightless existence. A solitude where no one else can reach me. A place where I can live for an eternity. Beneath my mother's beating heart, comforted by its steady rhythm. And it is only there that I can prepare myself to enter the world again.

Maybe that growing understanding explains why I *don't* fight the depression this time around. I just settle into the fetal position and listen for my mother's heartbeat.

Problem is, no matter how hard I listen, I still don't hear it. And then an even darker depression envelops me. I drop out of the Oriental Medicine program. I begin composing an email to Xavier to tell him I've had enough. That the trip back East has taught me that I no longer have a reason to heal. The truth is that no one has ever cared for me. And that no one ever will care for me. And worst of all, that I no longer have anyone to care for.

I guess I'm trying to prepare myself for an insulin dagger that will end it all. And for the first time in months I get down on my knees, reach into the farthest corner of the fridge and actually handle the vials of insulin. I hold them and wonder if they'll still do the trick.

But just holding them seems to be enough. So, I go back to my computer and pick up where I left off in my email to Xavier. *Life really sucks*, I write. Not sure if this really follows from what I wrote before. And the funny thing is that it feels *good* to write that life sucks. To let all that dark energy move through me and out of me. To release all that sadness and hopelessness and fury.

Fuck email, I decide. I'll call him.

Chapter Eighty-Four

"YOU KEEP MAKING the same mistake," says Xavier, after I tell him what's going on. "A decade's worth of steroids has eaten away at your powers of reasoning. And your ego, seeing its chance, is trying to take advantage. Trying to convince you, in your weakened state, that life isn't worth living."

I can't argue with that. As a nurse I know what long-term steroid use does to the body. *And* to the mind. And my doctors know too. And so does Rob. And yet whenever I'm feeling down he tells me to take them.

Just in case.

"The time has come," says Xavier, "for you to learn how to separate your actions from the actions of those around you."

"But what if I don't want to separate myself? Or isolate myself?"

"That's just your ego talking, not you. Just your ego taking advantage of your withdrawal from the drugs . . ."

". . . they're medications, *not* drugs."

"Call them what you want," he says, "but try this simple exercise." This can't be good. "Are you sitting down?" he asks me.

"Yes, I'm sitting down."

"Okay. List the things that are bothering you. The things that are really eating away at you."

Now it's my turn to take a deep breath. "How much time do we have?" I ask him.

277

"Don't fool around," he responds. "Stay focused."

"Okay," I say, taking a deep breath. "Knowing that my own family doesn't give a shit about me is one of the things that's really eating at me."

"Good," he says. "Now ask yourself, is that their problem, or yours? Or, to put it another way, ask yourself if that's *me*, or *not me*?"

"I don't have any idea what you're talking about."

We go back and forth for a while, and then he finally asks me the question that changes the way I look at everything.

"Your family doesn't give a shit about you, right?" he says. "*Me, or not me?*"

I have to think for a moment. "*Not me.*"

"That's right. Now give me another."

Suddenly the possibilities don't seem so endless. In fact, I have to think. "My fear that I'll be alone for the rest of my life."

"Good. *Me*, or *not me*?"

I don't really have to think about the answer. I just don't want to say it out loud. But I do. "*Me.*"

"Good. Now give me another."

I'm beginning to understand the game. "My children drinking themselves to death."

"Excellent example. *Me*, or *not me*."

"*Not me*. But I can still care, can't I?"

Chapter Eighty-Five

WITH DR. B.'s approval, I stop taking Levoxyl for my hypothyroidism. A few days afterward my blood tests show surprisingly normal levels of thyroid-stimulating hormone. And the question Xavier asked me months ago comes to mind.

What if none of it's true?

Which means there's nothing left but the steroids, as crazy as that seems. To me anyway. I guess I never really imagined it to be possible. Even after all my work with Xavier, a part of me still doesn't think it's possible.

Or maybe it's the *not me* who doesn't believe.

As if to prove the point, Rob arrives unannounced on the island, almost as if he were a shepherd trying to drive a stray back into the flock. I haven't seen him in four weeks. Since we'd come back from our trip to the East Coast.

Okay, so I *had* emailed him, and asked him to come. To help me through the process of weaning my body off the steroids. He never even responded.

Not me.

When I did hear from him it turned out that he had decided it was more important to attend a colleague's wedding. "It *was* important. There were more than four hundred people there," Rob told me over the phone. "The biggest names in the business."

Was I being unreasonable, asking him to be with me while I dealt with the withdrawal from the steroids? I don't know. Maybe, maybe not. But him not coming was *not me*. My asking, on the other hand, was *me*.

With Xavier's support, Dr. B. and I decide that I'd try going a couple days without Dexamethasone, the most powerful mind-altering medication I'd been given after Rob diagnosed my Addison's. I'd gotten through three days when Rob finally arrived. This time I haven't been counting the hours.

I know now that I have a choice. A real choice. After decades of living as if I didn't. It's what my parents taught me.

Not me.

It's what everyone taught me.

Not me.

What my siblings and my friends and my teachers and even my ministers taught me.

Definitely *not me.*

But what I accepted.

Me.

In their world, there was only one path for a woman. And that was to become dependent on a man. So even when I got my nursing degree, it was understood that my career was just a backup plan. In case my husband died or left me, and I was forced to support myself. Add to that the social capital of marrying a doctor, and the years of increasing wealth, and it was becoming easier and easier to understand why I'd clung to Rob so tenaciously. I'd been *taught* that I couldn't live without him.

Not me.

Finally seeing that I have a choice, I somehow get through the first week. Which I hope is worst of the withdrawal. And I do it all on my own.

The seventh day starts out as a gray sort of morning. Bleak but not ashy. By mid-morning, partly out of boredom and partly out of habit, I start the easy descent into self-pity. Then I do something that for me at least almost qualifies as superhuman.

I choose *not* to descend into depression.

Instead, I make myself a juice. I follow it with a bowl of quinoa and blueberries and almonds, and a splash of coconut oil.

I wander out to the patio and stand over my plants. Water them, and send them all the light and love I can. Okay, I'm still a little shaky. Might not have that much light and love to give at the moment. But it's the thought that counts. And we get what we give, right?

For once, though, I keep it simple. No melodrama. No demand for attention. Instead, I simply give thanks. For everything. For the bay. For the mountains. For my dog Beatrice. For the Omega-shaped scar Buddha inadvertently left on my calf. I give thanks for the sunshine and the salt air. I gave thanks to all my doctors back in California, even if they were so focused on treating my symptoms that they ignored the many possible causes of my illnesses.

I give loving thanks for my wayward children. For the way they're hanging in there as best they can. And perhaps just a little more reluctantly, I give thanks for my husband. Without him I wouldn't have a family. And then I really dive off the deep end and give thanks that my family is falling apart. I trust that something better will rise from the rubble. And then I end by giving thanks to my body, for putting up with me all these years. For hauling my aching spirit through this difficult life.

Wonderfully at peace, I email Xavier that I've had a great day, despite the physical discomfort of getting through it without steroids.

Steroids. My most powerful crutch. Along with drama.

But today I've taken care of *myself*. Just the way Xavier taught me.

It's a tremendous breakthrough. A spiritual breakthrough, as if the storm clouds have parted and I am bathed with light. As if I'd been walking through the desert and had finally come upon an oasis. Trusting all along that I would.

For the rest of the day I engage in radical self-care, delighting in each experience. I'm so proud of myself I can't stand it. Then I check my email. There's a response from Xavier.

> Credit? You want credit? Think about it. That's what got you into this mess in the first place. Your endless need for external validation. In order to truly heal, you have to learn to be satisfied with your own assessment of yourself. Not seek the praise of others.

My good mood dissolves like a drug in saline. I do the one thing you're not supposed to do when you're angry. I pick up the phone, full of self-righteous piss and vinegar. "I think I deserve *some* validation," I say when he picks up the phone. "I've worked really hard at this."

Xavier laughs. Which only fuels my anger. Like he's making fun of me. Treating the past seventeen months like some kind of a joke. And for the first time ever, he makes me think of Rob. Another one of those strong men who I had turned to for help, and who had laughed at my pain.

"What makes you think *you* deserve the credit for healing, anyway?" Xavier asks me. "*You* didn't do anything."

He's been telling me this from the beginning, but obviously, I still don't get it.

There is nothing for *me* to do. Healing isn't *my* job. My job is to create conditions conducive to healing.

"When you scrape your knee," he told me very early on, "you don't actually *do* anything to heal it. The scab forms on its own. The body knows how to repair itself without any help from you. The only thing you are required to do is keep the wound clean and *leave it alone*. Because if you pick at it, it will never heal."

Chapter Eighty-Six

I'VE BEEN OFF Dexamethasone for two weeks. I'm getting through the days, but my cortisol levels are still low. So at Rob's suggestion, over the phone, I supplement my natural steroids with Prednisone. It's a step backward, I know. But just one *small* step backward, after so many steps forward. And I can *feel* my body getting stronger. I can feel it aligning itself more with essence. Achieving health and wellness. And mindful of my small part in this, I concentrate only on giving my body sustenance. And the time it needs to rest. To adjust. To relearn how to depend on itself again.

A week later my cortisol levels are still low. But who knows what that really means? The drugs I had been taking for years *suppressed* my natural production of cortisol. So the only way to know for sure how much my body can produce is to get off the Prednisone too.

But just thinking about that causes anxiety to well up in me.

Not me.

Just the effect of quitting the medications, after so many years.

Not me.

I'm hanging on by my fingernails, I know. But I am hanging on.

When we take synthetic steroids, our brains no longer send orders to our adrenals. So the body becomes dependent on the external supply. The real question, therefore, is whether my adrenals will be able to resume their job when I quit taking synthetic steroids. And this is a real danger, not an imagined one. Especially because I'm alone so much of the time, and with low cortisol levels it's hard to think clearly.

Will I be able to care for myself? To feed myself? To call an ambulance if I have to?

Rob is on the mainland so I call Xavier. "Julie, we've been over this before," he says patiently. "You're addicted to drugs, so of course you're going to come up with some rationalization for continuing to take them."

"Well, they've kept me alive all these years," I tell him. "And if you want to call that a rationalization, then go ahead."

"And you're still addicted to drama, too, I see."

Shit. Is he right? Am I still a drug-addicted drama queen?

Me?

"Pain and illness," Xavier continues, "are simply invitations. They *invite* us to turn inward, to listen to the rhythm of our own hearts. They compel us to stop running. To stand still so we can reconnect with essence. This is the longing of every soul. To establish and reestablish its connection with essence. Over and over again. To look into the mirror and be able to smile and say, 'Oh, there you are. I've found you again.'"

Without the Dexamethasone, the mornings are the worst, because it stays with you twenty-four hours a day. Prednisone, instead, covers your needs for about eight hours. Which means that without the Dexamethasone I'm running on empty every morning. And my whole body aches. My joints hurt. I cry continually.

The nights aren't much better. I have drenching night sweats. A rapid pulse. My body swells as it works to flush out all the toxins. I feel like I'm nauseated all the time. Xavier advises me to eat every three hours. But my body rejects food. So he comes over and we do Qigong together. Which relaxes me a little. I can feel the energy moving through me again.

Encouraged, I cut back on the Prednisone. Use Cortef only to supplement. And Xavier calls me at least once a day. Reminds me that getting off synthetic steroids is an organic process. But that if I stick with it, my need for them will diminish. And then, in the same way I finally stopped needing the insulin, I'd simply forget to take the steroids one day.

Chapter Eighty-Seven

FOUR DAYS WITHOUT Prednisone. I feel a little unbalanced. Sick to my stomach. I try to eat every few hours to keep my blood sugar up. My body feels like a machine whose gears need oil. I sleep on the couch in the living room rather than in my bedroom. It's more open. There are more possibilities there. My bedroom is too much like a cave. I can't catch my breath in there.

Five days without Prednisone. My head spins. I sweat. My thoughts are scattered. Hard to hold on to. I remind myself that the goal is not to hold on but to let go. To watch my thoughts fleeing my body. Like I'm watching a movie.

But the movie makes no sense. The frames are blurred. I can't make out faces. Dialogue is slurred. I close my eyes and try to lie still as random thoughts continue to swirl around me. I feel my body pull energy in through the palms of my hands. The soles of my feet. My back.

"This is a surplus of yang," Xavier explains. "Anger, worry, and anxiety are all yang energies, and they're running rampant through your system, overwhelming your yin."

I nod my head. Barely able to listen, much less understand.

"Yang energy is hot and active, and like a fever it's overheating your system. So what you need are foods with cooling effects."

"Like what?" I ask.

"Oh, I don't know. Juice, perhaps?" he says.

Just what I need. Sarcasm.

"It's time to push yourself off the ocean floor and float," he says. "To trust that life will support you, and that the currents will take you where you need to go. And there's nothing for you to do but allow that to happen. Except to nourish yourself, of course, and to clear spaces in your heart and your mind so that trust and relaxation can find homes in you."

"And, of course," I add wearily, "love myself unconditionally."

Whenever I get my bearings for a moment, I try calling my children. Calling Rob. But no one answers. Unmoored and floating, I reach for the only thing I know, my old life. My family. Friends. Old habits. Even my illnesses. Any anchor I can think of.

Rob finally calls. "I don't see what the big deal is," he says, sounding like he's in a rush. "If you don't feel well, take some steroids."

I can't believe that I'm still hearing that from him.

"Look, Julie, I've gotta run. But don't forget, you're still the love of my life."

How many times have I longed to hear him say that? But even though it's probably withdrawal-induced paranoia, his saying it now convinces me that there's another woman.

Not me.

Eleven days without Prednisone. Sadness and restlessness envelop me. Curl their arms around me and squeeze me so tight it's hard to breathe. Consume so much energy that I'm not just tired, I'm exhausted.

I cry all the time.

I sleep without remembering my dreams.

Or maybe this is all a dream.

Fifteen days.

Xavier admonishes me to stop counting the days and to start living in the present. "The time has come," he tells me, "to let go of the past.

The days of illness and drugs are behind you. What you wanted to happen, has happened."

A life without illness and drugs.

Twenty days without Prednisone.

I cultivate stillness. Peace. A quiet house. No television. No radio. Just Beatrice and me. I write. I sleep. I eat. I allow my mind to come to rest.

And then, one day in the late summer of 2012, I am well.

All my lab work comes back normal. My adrenal production is back on line.

I can't believe it. It's a dream made real. If only my family were here to celebrate with me. But they aren't, and I understand why they're not. I'm the one who left to slay the dragon. And now that I've come back, the village is empty.

"We are all villages of one," says Xavier, "but the good news is that the sole inhabitant of your village is now well."

Chapter Eighty-Eight

SOON THEREAFTER, DR. B. dies unexpectedly in a skiing accident. I am devasted by the loss, and especially by what it must mean to his family. One of my children enters rehab. Another drinks to the point of blacking out. My marriage is falling apart.

What was the point of healing again?

"You tricked me," I complain to Xavier. "You tricked me into believing that life was worth living. You should have just let me die."

"Still addicted to drama, I see," said Xavier, indulging my tantrum.

I don't care what he says. Almost two years of hard work for nothing. Healing? What a crock of shit.

That evening I feel a fever spike. I'm warm to the touch. I have chills. I take my temperature and confirm the fever. I'm alone and I panic.

I hear Xavier's voice. *Be calm. Listen to your body.*

But I can't. Because I can't quiet the thumping of my heart. I offer my body food. It refuses.

I try some moxa. I try to meditate. But fear whispers in my ear. *If you're unable to help yourself, you'll die alone.*

I check my blood sugars. They're normal. I take my blood pressure. It's fine. But fear keeps me awake all night.

In the morning I drive myself to the emergency room. My lab work and EKG's are fine. There's nothing wrong with me. And for some reason this news infuriates me. Catapults me back in time to the year 2000, when my doctors still insisted that nothing was wrong with me. That I wasn't sick, just begging for attention.

Crazy, not sick.

"Take your blood pressure," Rob tells me when I call him.

All business. Playing the doctor. And assigning me the role of the patient. And what, after all, is more impersonal than the relationship between doctor and patient? It is in fact the foundation of the West's approach to medicine. The patient dependent on the doctor.

I take my blood pressure anyway.

"What is it?" he asks.

"It's 122 over 78," I tell him.

"Well," he says, "why don't you take a little Cortef. It can't hurt."

And then he's gone. Like a doctor hurrying off to the next exam room.

I reach for the Cortef bottle. But then I pause. Some part of me knows that if I open it, I'll be on the old merry-go-round again. So I just stand there for a moment. Step outside myself. Watch what's going on. And realize again that I have a choice.

I do not "have" Addison's disease. Or diabetes. Or hypothyroidism. Or Crohn's or cancer or any of the other Western diagnoses assigned me to appease my need for attention. My need for love. I have a hereditary disease instead. A pattern of self-destruction rooted in an inability to love *myself*. A pattern of behavior that can't be treated from the outside, because the cure, just like the root cause, exists within. Even if the diseases it creates are real.

With the Cortef bottle still in one hand, I reach for the phone to call Xavier. But it seems like the thought of calling him is all I need now. That is, to know that I don't *need* to call him. Because I already know what he'll say.

"Go make yourself some juice. Nourish yourself. Give yourself the attention you need. Stop expecting others to heal you. And stop creating drama. It distracts you. Just care for your body, and love yourself unconditionally."

It sounds so easy.

And for just a moment, it is.

Chapter Eighty-Nine

I 'M DRUG-FREE FOR nearly two months. Which is kind of funny since I used to think that what I wanted was to be illness-free. Now I'm just happy to be free of *all* of it.

To feel well.

I continue to write and to draw and to practice yoga and Qigong. Xavier continues to give me acupuncture and massage treatments. He tells me I should give Aikido a try.

Maybe in my next life.

I continue to nourish my body with juices and whole foods. I've started to gain more muscle mass. To look less fragile. Rob still flies over on occasion. Cole and Cat still stop by now and then. But the bonds that held us together have frayed. In fact they might be beyond repair, and I'm starting to be able to accept that. On most days. I accept that this is how things have to be.

In the meantime we're just playing at being a family. And we all know it.

But it's all right because it's all we can do right now. And something new is ready to be born. I can feel it kicking inside me. Letting me know it wants out.

I grow stronger every day, but I'm still occasionally blindsided by little bouts of sadness and anxiety. Even depression. Still, who in my position, wouldn't be? I've been a daughter and a wife and a mother. And a chronically ill patient and a drug addict. I've been a drama queen too. I've contemplated suicide.

But I am none of those women now.

"You're doing much better, but you're still reaching," says Xavier. "Whatever's coming will come in due time."

"You don't happen to have a schedule handy, do you?"

He shakes his head and smiles. Perhaps thinking about what I looked like more than a year and a half earlier.

"You know what happens when you reach for a leaf floating in a pool of water?" he asks me.

I shrug, not knowing or caring what the answer is.

"The disturbance you create by *touching* the water pushes the leaf farther away," he says. "So, if you want the leaf to come to you, stop reaching for it. It's really very simple."

Chapter Ninety

MY FATHER DIES.

It is November 2012, more than two years since I embarked on my journey of healing. Xavier would call it my ongoing journey. With a destination that is still unknown.

I am in London when the phone rings. It's my first trip out of the country since I weaned myself off my medications. I'm looking out our hotel window at the park below. The streetlights glow beneath halos of fog.

Rob and I are here together to see Cat. She's studying abroad for a semester.

A couple of months earlier, Rob and I began to talk about a trial separation, although I'd like it if we could remain friends. Maybe we could find a way to put the last thirty years behind us and start building something new.

What, exactly, I can't say. But if it's coming, it will come.

The years have left both of us bruised. Rob tells me I'm still the love of his life. I can't see how that could be true. Not given all the other women.

He still denies it, of course. But those weren't Cat's panties in his suitcase.

The truth is that I've changed so much he doesn't even really know me anymore. And the love of his life couldn't possibly be someone he doesn't know.

'Til health do us part.

It isn't even my phone that rings that morning in London. It's Rob's. My mother is calling with the news of my father's passing. Calling my husband. Not me. I feel anger tugging at me like a brush caught in my hair. But I remember to breathe. To allow the brush to move through my hair.

Like my relationship with Rob, my relationship with my mother will never change. It's frozen in time. Immobile in the rock hard but clear amber of our past. She still believes that I struck gold by marrying a doctor. The rest is meaningless. Yes, my healing was nothing short of miraculous. But now that I have done it, I'm supposed to go back to living the American Dream. Or at least her version of it. And give God sole credit for my recovery.

But of course I can't. And more importantly, I don't even want to try. Essence tells me to dismiss the challenge, and to focus on being mindful. And doing that, I think back to something my father told me a few weeks earlier. When we'd last talked on the phone. "You know, Julie, you're mine. You always have been, and you always will be."

I know now that I am not. Despite the many ways that both he and Rob tried to claim me.

Love without conditions. The heartbeat of the universe. Love that embraces everything. Without judgment or criticism. Love that gathers and nourishes and allows everything. But without any expectations. Love that tears down walls and sweeps aside veils. Love that restores sight, allowing us to see the universe with compassion. Love that heals even the deepest wounds.

If we can find the courage to allow it in, and receive its healing gift.

Chapter Ninety-One

Y OU SHOULD HAVE seen Aliceanne's face when she and I ran into each other at a gas station in Kailua in the fall of 2012. I was standing at the back of my car, one hand on the nozzle, waiting for the tank to fill when she pulled in behind me. I recognized *her* immediately. But she just glanced at me as she got out, then walked to the pump.

"Hey, Aliceanne."

She turned to face me, then squinted. If she knew me, she couldn't put a name to my face.

"It's Julie, Aliceanne," I said with a smile.

Her eyes opened wide. "Julie?"

I nodded. She looked at me for a moment longer, still unable to believe her eyes, then hurried over and gave me a long, heartfelt hug.

She wasn't the only one who didn't recognize me. Over and over again people I knew who haven't seen me since I healed would walk right past me, without a flicker of recognition. The change was that complete. Only my family and my friends Sherry and Lisbet had seen me as I healed. Everyone else simply couldn't believe it.

Including my doctors.

My endocrinologist, who had played the lead role in managing my care over the ten years following my Addison's diagnosis, didn't say a word when I walked into her office. Not at first anyway. She just got up from behind her desk, walked around, and put her arms around me without speaking. Then, holding me out at arm's length, she said, "I am so sorry, Julie."

My endocrinologist was the only member of my medical team who ever apologized to me. Although to be fair, I never needed to see most of the others again. Not after my year and a half with Xavier.

Not me.

As a nurse, I knew that my doctors had only done what 20th-century medical practice demanded of them. They'd written up patient histories. Performed physical examinations and had blood work done. Prescribed medications, which were followed by more exams and more lab work. And I asked them to do it. I was an enthusiastic patient, always eager to accept treatment. To discuss my latest symptoms and my body's reaction to the latest round of medications. To be the center of medical attention.

Me.

Like Liam said, I was never so happy as when I got a new diagnosis. Which meant I was a pretty happy girl back then. At first, anyway. Until my medical team prescribed so many medications that the interactions of the drugs, and their side effects, began to create health issues equally as serious as the diseases for which they'd been prescribed.

And yet, not once did any of them ask themselves if there might be another way. Nor, to be fair, did I. Not even when it was clear that their way wasn't working. We all did what we had been taught to do and never asked ourselves if the treatments might be doing more harm than good. Or if there might be something at work that a blood test couldn't detect.

Like emotional malnutrition.

"Hearts never really break," Xavier often reminds me. "They break *open.* And when they do, we can rid ourselves of things that no longer serve us. Create space for the new things to come."

Or, as he put it, we can't hold on *and* let go at the same time.

"It's really very simple. Just remain grateful, and maintain a healthy diet, because you're creating new cells every second. Which means that over time your body will totally recreate itself. Old cells die, and new cells are born, and all of those cells have memories. So, don't allow your new cells to share the same memories as your old cells, or you will never be able to heal completely."

"I can't even remember what I did yesterday, so I don't see how my cells are going to."

He shakes his head at me, but can't keep from smiling. "Just remember what you've learned," he says. "If you do, you'll not only continue to heal yourself, you'll heal the whole universe."

Afterword

In the first chapter of this book, which describes events that took place more than eight years ago, in the summer of 2010, I meant it when I said I couldn't take it anymore. And I'll bet every single person who lives with multiple chronic illnesses has felt like that way at one time or another. You just wish you could die. And in fact, some of my friends believed I went to Hawaii to do just that. To die peacefully, in a serene place.

But as I found out, dying is much harder than you think. And as usual, Xavier put it best. "The body is a self-correcting mechanism," he said. "If you feed yourself properly, and love yourself without conditions, your body will work as hard as it can to live."

Given where I am now, I'm very grateful that mine did.

Much has happened since I healed.

In November of 2012, my father died and I shaved my head and went to India. When I got back, Rob joined me on Oahu. While he was there, I did something I'd never done before. I began to search his devices. And sure enough, I found a series of incriminating texts. And photographs of women, too.

"Somebody else must have used my iPad," he said.

Sure. Right after they slipped out of their black panties and stuffed them into a pocket of your suitcase.

Not me.

We flew back to California to see our family therapist together.

"If you want to get through this," he told us, "you've both got to be honest."

Rob, it turned out, *was* prepared to be honest. Just not with me. He made an appointment to see our therapist alone the next day, and showing utter disregard for the rules, I followed him there. When I walked in and confronted him, he finally admitted everything. "I've been sleeping with other women."

I wasn't surprised. But it's one thing to suspect your husband is cheating on you, and another to hear him admit it out loud. And in front of someone else, too.

"How did it feel," I asked him, "to sleep with other women while your wife was in and out of the hospital, more dead than alive?"

He thought about it for just a moment. "Well, the sex was really good."

I stared at him. Didn't see a sign of remorse on his face. No guilt whatsoever. No sadness, and no apology.

"I think it's time I found myself a lawyer," I told him, and walked out.

Me.

It may sound hard to believe at this point in my story, but before I healed I had never once considered divorce. And I mean not *once* during the ten or eleven years of my chronic illnesses. I was just too sick. And even if I had given it any thought, I would never have followed through with it. I couldn't break up our family while the kids were still young. Besides, back then almost all my energy was directed toward managing my illnesses, and whatever was left went to the kids. So, it was only after I had healed physically that I was able to face up to the emotional malnutrition that was at the heart of all my problems.

And to finally deal with it.

Me.

I filed for divorce in the spring of 2013.

I think the kids knew it was coming. Maybe they even knew that it was the best thing for their father and me. If not necessarily for all of us.

Most of the people I knew who got divorced moved right into other relationships. In fact, most of the divorces I heard about resulted from one spouse having a relationship outside the marriage. And after moving out, the husband or the wife moved right back in, but with the other woman or the other man.

I can't speak for Rob, but I'm the only person I know who filed for divorce and then moved in with herself.

I stayed in Hawaii while the lawyers and the investigators went about their cruel business. I cried all the time, even though I knew I couldn't stay married to a man who had had ongoing relationships with other women for years, and who didn't want to give them up. Even while I was getting more and more sick. But knowing it was the only thing to do didn't make the breakup any less devastating. Why, I asked myself again, had I wanted to heal? So I could go through this?

The answer appeared to be yes. It finally became clear to me that for more than a decade, Rob and I had been bound together in *sickness*. My illnesses, which had made me a ward of the Western medical establishment, were the only things keeping Rob and me together.

'Til health do us part.

The next day I gathered all the insulin in the back of the fridge and threw it out.

A divorce requires almost as much energy as healing does. But if Xavier taught me anything, it's that you have to reduce unnecessary demands on your personal energy to make progress as a human being. And since the emotional demands of my failed marriage would *never* have ended, I asked my lawyers to go to work and then juiced my way through the long, heartbreaking process. I did my best to stay centered, as hard as that was given everything that was going on around me. Tried to let the kids' criticisms move right through me as best I could, instead of absorbing their anxiety and anger and storing it.

Of course to Xavier, all this was evidence that the universe was giving me new opportunities to grow. Everything that was happening, and everyone I bumped into, had something to teach me. Something to offer. As long as I was prepared to receive it, and to learn from it. To be open to it.

The divorce decree was granted in the summer of 2014, and I thought then that I had finally put all of this behind me. But of course I hadn't. I was so overwhelmed as it was happening that I couldn't really make sense of it. I just kept running on faith and hoped for the best. Which meant that it was only *after* our divorce that I was finally able to face up to what it really meant. And to make peace with it. That is, to make peace with what my marriage had done to me and to my health. With the way Western medicine and modern pharmacology had made a victim of me.

With my husband's help, and mine.

It was around that time I decided that I just *had* to put the long story of my illnesses and my healing down on paper.

I'd been attending writing workshops for years, mostly for therapeutic reasons. You know, if you can write about what happened to you, then you can understand what happened, maybe even accept it. After regaining my health, however, and divorcing my husband, what I really wanted was to make my story available to other women. Even if mine is a story without an ending, because healing is a process, not a journey with a specific destination. Put another way, no one ever completely heals.

So in the end, writing this book became a part of the healing process, too. And just like healing, I didn't do it on my own. I was lucky enough to find a number of guides to help me through it. But all the hard work will have been worth it if just one wife and mother out there finds hope in my story. That is, if one person is able to hope that she too might heal herself one day, and in so doing heal the world.

I rarely see my doctors these days, and when I do, my labs continue to come back normal. And of course the labs don't lie. Yes, my body still occasionally flushes out the remains of the drugs I was on for so long, and I still have phantom pains from surgeries I endured more than ten years ago. My skin still gets a little patchy from time to time. But I remain drug-free and healthy.

When I was healing I didn't know how to fill the hours. But now, even though my days are no longer structured around pills and injections and doctor's appointments, I can't seem to find the time to do everything I'd like to. I moved back to the mainland in 2016, shortly after my beloved Beatrice died of liver failure. As sad as that made me, it seemed as if her spirit was meant to move on to help someone else.

I rented a place in San Francisco for a year or so, then sold the beach house on Oahu and bought a cozy Victorian row house in San Francisco's Inner Richmond. It's got high ceilings, lots of light, a corner fireplace, and a couple of cats who were just kittens yesterday. It's still hard for me to comprehend how fast all living things grow.

Golden Gate Park is four blocks to the south, and the Presidio is four blocks to the north. Cole is staying with me for the time being, after graduating with honors from USF and studying in Japan. Cat lives nearby and splits her time between learning to become an herbalist and earning a master's degree in integral psychology. Liam is married with two young sons. He practices law in Chicago, and lives on a farm about a half an hour south of the city. Nathan, who has a degree from the University of Colorado, is in a grad program for computer science. He lives with Rob, in the house we all lived in so many years ago. The house where I almost died.

I've got a little garden of my own in the city. Most of it's in pots, but strawberries, tomatoes, cucumbers and squash spill out of them, along with lettuce for salads and herbs for cooking. Zen yoga classes are only six blocks away, and there's a meditation program at the local church. The public library on my block also has a heart/mind meditation class on Tuesdays, and there's a great Thai massage place not far away. But best of all, there's a fantastic cold press juice shop just six blocks away. So I get a little exercise and don't have to clean the juicer.

Xavier laughs when I tell him. "Still looking for shortcuts, aren't you?"

I'm finally ready to bring my story to a close now, but before I do there's one last thing I think I should add. Something that happened one afternoon at my house on Oahu, a couple of years ago, just before I left the island for the mainland.

I was out on the lanai tending to my plants when the phone rang. I glanced at the number and didn't recognize it, but I answered the phone anyway.

It was a woman I'd never met, calling from New York. She was a psychologist named Lucille who told me she'd spent the last couple of weeks in the hospital with her dying mother. Her father, who had abused her terribly when she was younger, had passed away a year or so before. She was divorced and had raised her children alone. She was also a breast cancer survivor. And as if life hadn't been tough enough already, she had just been diagnosed with lung cancer.

"How did you get my number?" I asked her.

"Well," she said, "I know this is going to sound crazy, but a friend of a friend of mine in North Carolina somehow knew your whole story. You know, about how sick you were, and how you healed. And, well, I just couldn't get it out of my mind, especially with everything that was going on with me and my mom and my kids. So, it wasn't easy, but I finally tracked you down."

A brief silence followed.

"Anyway," she continued, "that was about a week ago, and today, well, I finally found the courage to call you."

I didn't know what to say. But she did. "Can you help me heal?"

A thousand things went through my mind, as if every day of my year and a half with Xavier was passing in front of my eyes again. What was I supposed to tell her? That she had to leave her toxic environment to heal? That she had to quit smoking and give up red meat and bread? Make herself a lot of fresh, easily digestible juices, and most importantly, find the courage to tell the universe that she loved herself unconditionally?

None of that sounded right coming from me.

What I really wanted to tell her was that even though I did heal myself, or at least got out of my body's way so it could heal itself, *I'm not a healer.* I'm just a woman who was very, very sick, and somehow found her way back to health. A woman who is *still* healing. But I couldn't just tell her that and hang up. Not after she'd heard my story and had gone to all the trouble to find me.

"Do you have a pen?" I asked her, thinking on my feet, "because I know a guy who's perfect for you. He's a Boston-born Eastern healer by the name of Xavier Staub. Vietnam vet, sixth-degree black belt in Aikido. Lives here on Oahu."

Now, if I ever get a phone call from another woman who's eager to hear my story, I can simply tell her about *'Til health do us part.* Which means that Xavier was right. By healing myself I have begun to heal the world. By caring for myself, I somehow touched the life of a stranger, a woman who lived six thousand miles away. A woman I'd never met. And yet somehow my story brought us together and brought her a measure of peace when she needed it most.

So it *is* true. We *can* heal ourselves and each other with our thoughts, our actions, and our stories, and in so doing we can heal the world. Almost as if the words I first spoke so many years ago, high above the Pacific Ocean on Lahilahi Point, are still echoing through the universe.

Acknowledgments

FIRST, I WANT to acknowledge all those who continued to love me through my illnesses *and* healing, especially Sherry, Lisbet, Ron, Francesca, Mary and Lucille. Just as importantly, I wish to acknowledge all those who could not love me, because *you* were truly my most effective teachers.

I also wish to acknowledge the multitude of writing angels who appeared with almost divine timing throughout this process, especially Aliceanne, Mark, Jen, Lisbet and Cory. Without you these words would never have made it to the page, and I would never have been able to heal fully.

I also want to acknowledge my children, the greatest gifts I have ever been given.

Finally, I want to acknowledge my guide, Xavier, who has never taken or accepted credit for my healing, and who continually encourages me to see that the credit is not mine, either. I am grateful for all of you, and wish you all health, happiness and understanding.